The
ART OF MEDICINE

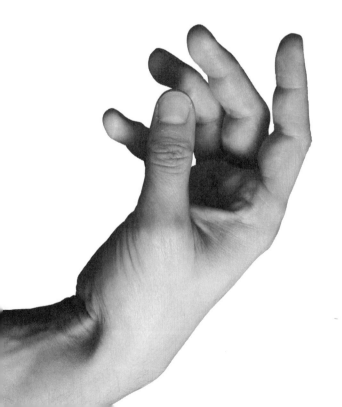

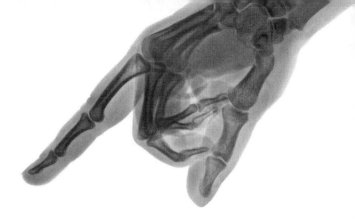

The
ART OF MEDICINE

HEALING *and the* LIMITS *of* TECHNOLOGY

DR. HERBERT HO PING KONG
with MICHAEL POSNER

ECW PRESS

Published by ECW Press
2120 Queen Street East, Suite 200, Toronto, Ontario, Canada M4E 1E2
416-694-3348 / info@ecwpress.com

LIBRARY AND ARCHIVES CANADA CATALOGUING IN PUBLICATION

Ho Ping Kong, Herbert, author
The art of medicine : healing and the limits of technology
/ Dr. Herbert Ho Ping Kong with Michael Posner.

Issued in print and electronic formats.
ISBN 978-1-77041-173-9 (bound)
Also issued as 978-1-77090-565-8 (PDF) and 978-1-77090-566-5 (EPUB)

1. Physicians. 2. Medicine. 3. Patient-centered health care.
4. Physician and patient. 5. Patients—Interviews. I. Posner, Michael, 1947–, author II. Title.

R727.3.H45 2014   610.69'5   C2014-901307-8
C2014-901308-6

Cover design: Michel Vrana
Cover images: Valeniker/Shutterstock, eAlisa/Shutterstock
Type: Rachel Ironstone
Printed and bound in Canada at Friesens   1   2   3   4   5

A note on the type: MVB Verdigris Pro was designed by Mark van Bronkhorst in 2003; it is a Garalde text face for the digital age, inspired by the work of 16th-century punchcutters.

The publication of *The Art of Medicine* has been generously supported by the Canada Council for the Arts which last year invested $157 million to bring the arts to Canadians throughout the country, and by the Ontario Arts Council (OAC), an agency of the Government of Ontario, which last year funded 1,681 individual artists and 1,125 organizations in 216 communities across Ontario for a total of $52.8 million. We also acknowledge the financial support of the Government of Canada through the Canada Book Fund for our publishing activities, and the contribution of the Government of Ontario through the Ontario Book Publishing Tax Credit and the Ontario Media Development Corporation.

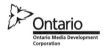

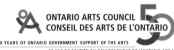

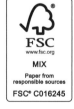

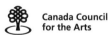

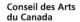

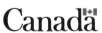

THIS BOOK IS DEDICATED TO

The Ho Ping Kong Family:

Dr. Barbara Ho Ping Kong

Christine, Peter, Roger, Wayne,

Cindy (children & their spouses)

Michael, Sarah, Abbe & Ian

(grandchildren) and the thousands

of patients, trainees and colleagues

who inspired me to write this book.

WE ACKNOWLEDGE THE GENEROUS

AND DEDICATED SUPPORT OF:

The Honourable G. Raymond Chang

Chancellor Emeritus Ryerson University

Foundation Board Member for Education

University Health Network, Toronto

and the Centre for Excellence in Education

and Practice (CEEP) at the University Health

Network, Toronto Western Hospital

TABLE *of* CONTENTS

FOREWORD

THE RELATIONSHIP BETWEEN A PHYSICIAN and patient is truly multidimensional. Dr. Herbert Ho Ping Kong captures this important concept in the opening chapter of *The Art of Medicine* when he emphasizes the art of seeing, listening, human touch, empathy, advocacy, recognizing suffering and thinking outside the box. Then, in his remarkable style of clinical narrative, Dr. Ho Ping Kong proceeds to interweave patients' stories with proverb, literary quotation and metaphor to illustrate the relevance of these arts as essential to effective medical practice.

Dr. Ho Ping Kong has dedicated his academic career to educating generations of students and residents in the art and science of internal medical practice. His influence has been indelible on all of us who have been privileged to work with him as trainees and clinical colleagues. I was thrilled to learn he was writing this book, which reflects not only Dr. Ho Ping Kong's unique teachings blending the art and science of medicine, but also the learning experiences of a number of our colleagues, some of them his former students, who share a passion for understanding the personal context of their patients.

One purpose of this book is to provide medical students, trainees and aspiring physicians with insight into the meaning of their profession — beyond the acquisition of technical and diagnostic competencies. All too often as medical students graduate and enter very busy residency programs and ultimately their own practices, they are caught up in the constant pressures of focussing on diagnosing and treating disease. The person who confronts them with illness may become less important to the doctor who is constantly constrained by lack of time, inefficient health care systems, language or cultural barriers — to name only a few challenges of daily practice.

Yet the challenge of seeing beyond the disease to the illness that affects a person is often of critical importance in making the right diagnosis and choosing the most effective therapeutic interventions. The mutual satisfaction of developing a relationship built on trust and respect experienced by both physician and patient underpins the most meaningful aspect of medical practice and the art of healing. Of particular interest, illustrated in this inspiring text, is that generalist and specialist practitioners describe the same approaches to the art of medicine, implying its universality.

Dr. Ho Ping Kong has created a rare window of opportunity for his colleagues to express their deepest held thoughts and beliefs about why and how they practise the art of medicine. These mini essays, interwoven through the text, provide other perspectives on the art of medicine, by physicians of diverse specialties. As Dr. Peter Singer says, communication and sensitivity can be taught to medical students. Leadership and judgment are perhaps more readily acquired through mentorship and role modelling as exemplified by Dr. Ho Ping Kong.

But this is not only a book for the medical community. Ordinary consumers — users of the health care system — will glean many insights from the analysis of his cases and his views on the critical nexus of technology and patient-centred medicine.

On behalf of all who read and are inspired by this book, I sincerely thank the contributors, and Dr. Ho Ping Kong in particular, for sharing their wisdom and knowledge about the art of medicine — an enduring lesson for all of us.

Catharine Whiteside, M.D., Ph.D.
Dean of Medicine
University of Toronto
February 2014

FOREWORD

WHAT IS THE ART OF MEDICINE? It is a concept which is often hard to define, but which is easy to recognize. In his daily clinical practice as a general internist, Dr. Ho Ping Kong (HPK) embodies this art. I am one of his junior colleagues in the Division of General Internal Medicine and have had many opportunities to observe him and to learn from him. As someone with a graduate degree in the social sciences, I sought to explore and understand the different components of the art of medicine, and to make concrete the ineffable qualities that HPK incarnates as a clinician. In this foreword, I will share some of the components of this evanescent art. Paradoxically, one of the ways in which I came to think about the art of medicine was to invert the phrase itself and to put forward a new trope to define our roles as clinicians: the physician-as-artist. I suggest that as health care providers who practise the art of medicine, we are not simply automatons who implement algorithms. Undoubtedly, we must integrate our knowledge about medical sciences into our practices. But the concept of physician-as-artist forces us to recognize, teach and account for all of the other aspects of our clinical work that HPK intuitively knows and demonstrates. Through this trope, I will describe how the art of medicine encompasses and celebrates practitioners who are creative, imaginative, responsive and compassionate.

The physician-as-artist is CREATIVE *and* IMAGINATIVE. Physicians must learn to think laterally — to think outside the box as well as within it. Creative thinking engenders novel therapies and novel health care delivery solutions. Physicians think creatively when trying to elucidate a diagnosis in a patient who has a disparate constellation of symptoms. We think creatively when we challenge the status quo and innovate — whether in clinical care, clinical education or health systems reform. The physician-as-artist is also able to imagine herself as a patient, just as an actor in the Royal Shakespeare Company may don Prospero's robe and imagine himself as a magician. What is it like to be hospitalized, to be immobilized, to be confused or to be in pain? How does a patient's particular cultural, personal, social or family history influence their illness experience?

The physician-as-artist is AWARE *and* RESPONSIVE. As physicians, we should be sensitive and perceptive to our own surroundings and to those of our patients. We should recognize and respond to the physical, the emotional and psychological well-being of our patients. This multidimensional model of health is a characteristic that HPK exemplifies and promotes. I suspect that it is one of the reasons why his patients seek to visit him routinely even when they are no longer ailing. He always asks questions about life beyond the physical illness — about families, jobs, travels, joys and sorrows.

The physician-as-artist is AFFECTIVE *and* EMBODIED. A physician has emotions. Most health care practitioners can recall difficult, frustrating, saddening or fulfilling encounters with patients or their families. To invoke an idea described by my friend and scholarly mentor, social scientist Natasha Myers, we must recognize that we *move with* and are *moved by* our patients.[1] Furthermore, during medical school and residency, we entrain our bodies in addition to our minds. Although this process is most obvious for surgeons who learn the physical skills of cutting and suturing, it applies similarly to internists. Just as an artist articulates her senses or learns her physical craft, physicians learn procedures, train our ears to distinguish heart sounds and our hands to discern masses or nodes. Physicians should not be emotionally disengaged and disembodied scientific minds. We must pay attention to our own emotions, senses and physicalities in order to attend to those of our patients.

The physician-as-artist has PERSPECTIVE. The notion of having a *situated* perspective rather than an all-seeing and omniscient one highlights one of the major paradigm shifts in 20th-century thought.[2] It represents the transition from modernism, in which the truth and objectivity of scientific knowledge were assumed, to postmodernism, in which a multiplicity of truths is recognized. Thus, no matter how objective or removed from its object of study a scientist or physician may be, he always has a situated perspective — one which depends on politics, culture, race, socioeconomic status, etc. Rather than having our physician identities subsumed by a stethoscope (a tool which evolved to both literally and figuratively distance a physician from patients and perhaps even from herself as person), the concept of physician-as-artist draws to attention the individual perspectives that we bring to our practices. In enacting his own art of medicine, HPK simultaneously melds therapies based on medical evidence with experiential knowledge arising from his own perspectives and those of his patients.

TO HELP DISCERN THE ART of medicine, I have put forward the simile of physician-as-artist. The physician-as-artist thinks creatively; attends to his own perspectives, emotions and physicality; and listens for, imagines and reflects on the perspectives of others — most notably those of her patients. All of these qualities underscore one of the most fundamental components of physicianship: caring. This quality is one which HPK truly exemplifies. It is a quality which will weave together the chapters in this book as we seek to further understand the art of medicine.

Dr. Lisa Richardson
Division of General Internal Medicine,
University of Toronto
February 2014

1   Myers, Natasha. 2007. *Modeling proteins, making scientists: an ethnography of pedagogy and visual cultures in contemporary structural biology*. Ph.D. dissertation, MIT.

2   Haraway, Donna J. 1991. *Simians, Cyborgs and Women: The Reinvention of Nature*. New York: Routledge.

PREFACE

"HOW ARE YOU FEELING?" Dr. Herbert Ho Ping Kong asked me.

We were sitting in one of our weekly meetings in his corner office. I wasn't his patient at the time; I was conducting an interview for the project that would become this book. It was a question he usually asked as a matter of course and, on this particular winter morning, I was hoping he would ask again.

The truth is, I had lately been experiencing bouts of what I thought was angina pectoris — chest pain — caused by blockages in the arteries of the heart. When I climbed even a short hill, I began to feel an uncomfortable tugging. At first, I thought it must be muscle pain, related to lifting weights in the gym. But muscle pain normally subsides after a few days. This pain persisted over several weeks and had begun to trouble me.

I have a long family history of heart disease. My late father had suffered his first heart attack at age 48. Several of his siblings had been stricken as well. My own electrocardiograms ostensibly showed no evidence of trouble, but these, I later discovered, had been misread.

For several days, I had wrestled with the decision of whether to raise my concern with Dr. Ho Ping Kong. The proper route was to see a general practitioner and solicit a referral to a cardiologist. On the other hand, the holiday season was upon us and I feared I'd have to wait weeks for an appointment. I thus felt conflicted, knowing the protocol and not wanting to jump the queue, but also increasingly anxious about my health.

So when he inquired about my health that day, I spoke up. Dr. Ho Ping Kong then asked a few pointed questions about my pain — when I experienced it, how long it lasted. He then rose from his chair, left the room and returned a few minutes later to advise me that I'd be seeing his partner, cardiologist Dr. John Janevski, the next morning at 8 a.m. for a series of tests.

The news at the end of that day was not encouraging. I had effectively failed the treadmill stress test. Worse, Dr. Janeski's more careful reading of two old electrocardiograms indicated that I had already suffered one minor heart attack, probably five years earlier.

A fortnight later, I underwent an angiogram, an injection of contrasting dye into the heart. The results were shocking to me. It found a 99 percent blockage in my main coronary artery, and 70 percent blockages in the next two largest. Diagnosed with so-called unstable angina, which meant I was liable to suffer another heart attack at any time, I was kept in the hospital and underwent triple bypass surgery four days later.

I was indebted to the teams of doctors and nurses who had acted promptly and with great skill to perform the necessary procedures. But in the first instance, I was particularly indebted to Dr. Ho Ping Kong. His alert response to my complaint, his ability to sense that something might indeed be wrong with my heart, very likely saved my life.

Of course, I already knew how fortunate I and his other patients are. Some years earlier, I had developed a strange set of other complaints, including aching limbs, low-grade fever, chills and crippling fatigue. My family doctor, ultimately stumped about the diagnosis, had sent me to see Dr. Ho Ping Kong.

After a series of meetings and a round of tests — blood work, x-rays, a spinal tap and a session with a psychiatrist to check for possible depression — he offered his best guest: polymyalgia rheumatica, an autoimmune disorder. It was his best guess because there is no definitive test for PMR. It's one of those Grey Zone diseases that are hard either to prove or disprove. I was started on a course of prednisone and worked my way through a reducing dosage for about a year. By that time, the symptoms had virtually disappeared.

By the time he suggested we work together on a book that would encapsulate his views on the art of medicine, I already knew that HPK, as he is widely known, was that rare combination of brilliance and sensitivity. My conviction only deepened during the following months of interviews, as I talked to his colleagues, his patients and some of his students.

I was also able to spend countless hours in his company, listening — fascinated — while he exhumed old cases from his inexhaustible memory and explained their importance. He worked from a large black diary book in which he had jotted down perhaps one seminal fact from a particular case, often just a name. And from that tiniest of takeoff points, he would then soar, expounding in minute detail the origin, evolution and final disposition of the case, including hemoglobin counts and heart rates — even if the case was 40 or 50 years old.

When I interviewed HPK's colleagues, I was struck by two predominant themes — a collective sense of awe about his diagnostic acumen and his ability to forge genuine, human relationships with his patients. Strikingly, the physicians regard the latter gift as no less important than the former. Many other physicians,

THE ART OF MEDICINE

they note, are often good at one or the other, but few demonstrate Ho Ping Kong's extraordinary facility in both. It represents a potent bedside combination.

As you make your way through this instructive memoir, I hope that you will share my feeling of how fortunate we are to have even a portion of his vast medical experience and timeless wisdom recorded for the next generations of physicians and patients alike.

Michael Posner

February 2014

INTRODUCTION

The practice of medicine is an art, not a trade; a calling, not a business; a calling in which your heart will be exercised equally with your head. Often the best part of your work will have nothing to do with potions and powders, but with the exercise of an influence of the strong upon the weak, of the righteous upon the wicked, of the wise upon the foolish.

— Sir William Osler

"SO, TELL US, DR. HO PING KONG, what do you think about our unit?"

The year was 1968. I was attending the regular Monday morning meeting of physicians at the Tropical Metabolism Research Unit, on the campus of the University of the West Indies in Kingston, Jamaica.

Set up by Britain's Medical Research Council, its focus was on childhood nutrition — particularly a disease with a very strange name, kwashiorkor, a form of malnutrition caused by lack of dietary protein — a serious concern in the Caribbean in the years that followed the Second World War. The importance attached to the unit was reflected in the physician named to be founder, the distinguished Dr. John Waterlow.

I was a third-year resident, a minor player. I was doing

research, a study — later published in the *Lancet* — on urinary acidification in adults with sickle-cell anemia.

The unit's senior scientist was nephrologist Dr. George Alleyne, a powerhouse in the Jamaican medical community and, later, on the world stage as a chairman of the Pan American Health Organization. Most of what Alleyne's Centre was doing was outside my principal areas of interest. But that morning, chairing the meeting, he had asked me a pointed question, and I had never been one to shy away from speaking my mind.

"Well," I began, "I'm not a nutritionist, so I'll confine my remarks to some observations about the ward. It's very clean, and the nurses are very efficient. But I think you are doing something wrong with the babies in those cribs. They don't laugh. They are lifeless . . . passive . . . inert. They have no animation. I think that's wrong. I think you should lift the restriction on nurses hugging the children. Maybe," I ventured, "you should hug them yourself."

The room fell quickly silent, clearly puzzled, if not shocked, by my candour. The colour drained from Dr. Alleyne's face. I knew I was right, but perhaps had overstepped the bounds of propriety. I left the meeting soon after.

I soon forgot about the incident, immersed as I was in a career that would eventually lead me away from my beloved Jamaica, to Montreal's Royal Victoria Hospital and McGill University, and later to Toronto's University Hospital Network, a constellation of world-class facilities that includes Toronto Western Hospital, Toronto General Hospital and the Princess Margaret Hospital. Years passed, during which my relationship with Alleyne remained friendly but distant. Although we would occasionally see each other, we never spoke about that day.

Fast forward some 40 years. A Jamaican friend, business-man Ray Chang — chancellor of Toronto's Ryerson University, a Toronto Western Hospital board member and a major philan-thropist — was honouring me with a gala dinner for my contribu-tions to medicine in Canada and the Caribbean. Alleyne, now the

University of the West Indies' chancellor, had been invited to say a few words and, braving a winter snowstorm, had travelled from Washington to Toronto for the occasion.

To my great surprise, he recounted the story of that morning meeting at the unit — of how I had brazenly dared to tell him and his staff that they were running a poor show. At the time, he conceded, he had been stung by my criticism. "Herbert doesn't even know how hurt we were," he said.

But, he continued, "Dr. Ho Ping Kong was right. The children did need to be touched and hugged." In fact, the following year, the Metabolic Unit hired Dr. Sally McGregor, a remarkable physician who would ultimately author some 150 papers on the emotional development of children with malnutrition. The importance of touching became a major theme in her work.

From whence did my youthful boldness derive? I'm not sure. I simply felt my opinions were well grounded, both in medical and humanistic terms.

Some years earlier, during my third year of medical studies, a group of about a dozen senior cardiologists and registrars was conducting rounds on the ward. Students weren't formally part of the team, but I had managed to position myself strategically within auditory reach to absorb whatever nuggets of medical wisdom that I could.

As it happened, one of the physicians, a professor of cardiology, noticed me lurking, summoned me to the patient's bedside and instructed me to listen to his heart. I was nervous, but not lacking confidence; I'd been on the cardiac ward for three months and had spent virtually every evening listening to murmurs on all the patients that would allow me to examine them.

I approached and applied the stethoscope and, after listening for perhaps 15 seconds, delivered my judgment.

"Sir," I said, "this is an early diastolic murmur. It's very soft, sir, but I think it's aortic incompetence."

"Listen again," he commanded.

So I listened for the second time and reached the same conclusion. "I think I'm correct, sir. The aortic valve is defective."

"What year are you in?"

"Third year, sir."

"You know, if you were wrong and you were in fourth year, I'd fail you."

"I'm pretty sure I heard it, sir."

One of the senior registrars then placed his stethoscope on the patient's chest.

"The student is right," he finally said. "This is an early diastolic murmur."

Perhaps it was that incident that gave me the courage of my diagnostic convictions. In the years since then, I have only rarely relinquished them.

For me, the case demonstrated a critical distinction — the difference between listening and hearing. Every doctor is trained to hear, but not every doctor is trained to listen, to detect the subtle distinctions in cardiac behaviour that may spell the difference between life and death.

Hearing is often passive and automatic. Listening implies a higher level of active engagement. When you truly listen to the heart sounds, for example, you can detect subtle but critical indications of the organ's health — loudness, character, the timing of its cycle, its radial signature and its relationship to breathing.

The same distinction applies to the acts of looking and seeing, as well as to the art of touch. It is not enough simply to touch the spleen or the liver. One must actually palpate the organs — determine the size, shape and consistency in relation to the surrounding organs and tissue.

THE PRACTICE OF MEDICINE IS generally considered a science. In fact, science itself has its roots in medicine. In the modern age, it is science that has taken humankind on our remarkable extended voyage of discovery about the body and the myriad illnesses to which it is prone. In the last century, that journey has been expedited by the increasingly complex machines that survey, map and analyze our veins and arteries, our organs and our brains.

I have now been engaged in the practice of medicine for almost five decades. During that time, I have witnessed extraordinary, almost miraculous changes — stunning advances in our knowledge of the mechanisms of disease; an exponential growth in our understanding of biochemistry; amazing developments in science and technology that have facilitated improved diagnosis, preventions and treatment. Many of these strides were made on the back of our spectacular breakthroughs in medical technology. Yet for all this, I submit, medicine — the word itself derives from the Latin *medicina*, meaning the healing art — remains as much an art as a science.

The wisest doctors know that science is not omniscient. The science of medicine has limits — and the often-arcane secrets of health and disease do not always yield to the microscope and the test tube, the MRI and the CT scan, the x-ray machine and the laproscopic probe.

Science itself is, by definition, provisional: our knowledge — the result of testing and retesting — stands until it is overtaken by superior knowledge. A good example, drawn from the world of medicine, is the stomach ulcer. For decades, it was medical consensus that ulcers were caused by poor diet or stress. Now, it is widely believed that at least 90 percent of all duodenal ulcers are caused by bacteria. In the final analysis, physicians know, many mysteries remain — conditions that produce symptoms that have no formal name, disease that has a name but no effective remedy. As the great physician and essayist the late Lewis Thomas once said, "The most solid piece of scientific truth I know of is that we are profoundly ignorant about nature."

Indeed, I would even argue that the more progress we make

on the scientific front — the more weapons we accumulate — the more critical the "art" part of the professional partnership becomes.

Among the range of talents needed to be used, perhaps nothing is more important than the human faculties — treating patients with compassion, understanding, empathy and solid clinical judgment. This book demonstrates why this is so.

WHAT EXACTLY DO I MEAN by "the art of medicine"?

I mean, in the first instance, a greater emphasis on the human factor — precisely the sort of humanity that I noticed was missing from the ward of the Tropical Metabolism Unit in Kingston.

I mean bringing three key human senses — sight, hearing and touch — more centrally into the doctor-patient relationship in prevention, diagnosis and treatment.

I mean learning how to become an advocate for patients, both within and without the medical community.

I mean bringing empathy, intuition, out-of-the-box thinking and attention to the entire patient — mind and body — to the bedside or examination table.

And I mean learning how properly to care for patients who cannot be helped, either because their condition is terminal or because, as we see more and more in modern times, we cannot attach a specific name to a specific set of medical complaints.

As complexity increases, and costs rise, and waiting times lengthen, and organizations grow, it has become harder and harder for patients to navigate through what often seems to be a confusing labyrinth — the modern medical system. In such circumstances, it is all the more essential that physicians supplement their vast database of knowledge with the human touch.

In the book that follows, I want to explore these issues from several vantage points — drawing lessons from the archive of my own 50-year dossier of cases; from the point of view of patients with whom I have dealt; and from my distinguished colleagues in Montreal and Toronto, who have their own valuable perspectives on how to add more value to care-giving.

I am writing, I hope, for a dual audience — the medical community at large, particularly the coming generation of young physicians, which must obviously bear the final responsibility for determining the future of clinical practice; and for the general public — patients — who perhaps can use the stories in these pages to seek and obtain higher, more humane standards of care. They need it — and they deserve it.

CHAPTER I

The ART
of MEDICINE

It is more important to know what sort of person has a disease than to know what sort of disease a person has.
— Hippocrates

METAPHORICALLY, THE ART OF MEDICINE is a clinic that contains many rooms. In each, a different art is demonstrated.

In one room, there is the art of seeing, diagnosing illness by carefully observing what may be hiding in plain sight.

In a second, there is the art of listening, actively tuning in to the signature rhythms of the patient's body, hearing both what the patient says and, equally important, what he or she may not be saying.

In a third, there is the art of human touch, which includes not only feeling the pulse, palpating the spleen, the kidneys and other organs to make the diagnosis, but may also include simply holding the patient's hand to let them know that you care.

Two other rooms are dedicated to what is often called the Grey Zone. One is for patients who exhibit a range of clinical symptoms that defy simple diagnosis. They are clearly suffering, but there is no agreed-upon name for their ailment. How does the sensitive clinician deal with that increasingly common situation?

The other Grey Zone room accommodates patients who have a definable illness for which there is no specific or reliable treatment. Here, again, the good physician must demonstrate the art of medicine through care management, always bearing in mind the ancient injunction *primum non nocere*: first, do no harm.

In a sixth room, there is the art of communication — how to elicit vital information, build trust, deliver bad news and inspire hope, even in the most adverse circumstances.

In a seventh room is empathy, understanding the context of any particular illness — its effects on the individual, their life and the lives of their extended families — and expressing that understanding to all concerned.

Another room is devoted to advocacy, asserting the patient's interests within the medical system and, if necessary, beyond.

There are other rooms as well, rooms for thinking outside of the box, treating rare diseases and dealing with epidemics.

For the sake of convenience, I am describing these salons as if they were discrete silos. The truth is otherwise. In fact, the doors to all these rooms connect and, in most situations, the doctor must travel back and forth between and among them, in his or her relentless search for the best answer.

In the process, the good clinician will wear many hats at once — healer, detective, adviser, scientist and artist, deploying the colours of a broad palette.

One must see, listen, touch, communicate, empathize, etc. — yes. But most of all, the challenge of the art of medicine is to integrate what is learned in each of the various rooms and synthesize that knowledge to find the right approach, if not always the perfect answer.

But for the art of medicine, one factor stands paramount: time. Time is the essential ingredient — time not only to win the patient's trust, but the time necessary to take a complete history, conduct a thorough physical exam and carefully consider all the diagnostic and therapeutic options. And time, in many instances, to allow nature to take its appointed course.

In this first chapter, I want to provide examples from my own case histories that illustrate a few of these aspects of the art of medicine in action.

ONE DAY IN TORONTO, AS I ACCOMPANIED a senior clinician and a junior internist on rounds, we encountered Giuseppe, an 80-year-old Italian who had been treated for cellulitis. However, he had recently developed some new skin lesions on his feet, an indication of infection, possibly the result of staphylococcus, potentially destructive bacteria. Still, the staff wasn't quite sure what was wrong.

We entered his room and found he had three visitors, his wife and two daughters. While my colleagues examined the patient, I made small talk with the family and learned that Giuseppe had been born in southern Italy and had immigrated to Canada many years earlier.

Eventually, I was asked to examine the small lumps on his feet, which were slightly purplish in colour, like blueberries.

"So what do you think?" my senior colleague asked me.

"I think it's probably going to be Kaposi's sarcoma," I said.

Since the early 1980s, Kaposi's sarcoma — named for the Hungarian dermatologist who first described it — has been most frequently associated with HIV/AIDS patients. That form of the illness is very aggressive, often and quickly spreading to the lungs, brain and the GI tract.

But there are several other variants of the disease, including one that historically affects elderly men of the Mediterranean region. I'd seen it before, perhaps two or three times. This strain of KS is less virulent. It can be treated with low-dose radiation, and death is rare.

My comment drew incredulous looks from the medical team. How could I make that diagnosis of a rare illness, based simply on a brief examination of his feet?

The answer was not complicated. It merely required me to integrate what I could plainly see — the "blueberries" on Giuseppe's feet — with my newfound knowledge of the family's history. Both pieces of information were equally vital.

A subsequent biopsy of Giuseppe's tissue confirmed my diagnosis. But again, it was the not-so-casual human interaction — talking to the family about his origins — that had given me the first clues.

SOMETIMES, THE ART OF MEDICINE in diagnosis is based as much on raw instinct as on evidence. Of course, raw instinct is not entirely raw; it's based on experience, for which there is ultimately no substitute. As one mordant Hindu proverb puts it, "No physician is really good until he has killed one or two patients."

One day, a former chief resident of mine, now working in another city, called and asked whether he could refer a case to me. The patient would not be coming for an office visit, so I would have to "examine" him by reading his medical dossier, which would be emailed to me. The patient was a 40-year-old Canadian who had served in Bosnia during the war and been injured. The injury had required a blood transfusion. His file indicated that he was suffering from fever, weakness and a low white blood cell count. Collectively, these symptoms suggested the possibility of HIV/AIDS, but a test for the disease had proven negative. Despite that negative reading, I wondered whether he might, in fact, have HIV/AIDS. I called my former colleague.

"I think you should redo the HIV test," I said.

"Why?" he asked. "He's negative."

"Yes, but he has the classic symptoms of that terrible wasting disease. And he underwent a blood transfusion." Tragically, many HIV/AIDS victims are infected through the transfusion process.

The test was re-administered and, this time, the result was positive. Sometimes, tests are improperly performed, skewing the outcome. Sometimes, the test is given before the disease is fully manifest, so it is missed. And sometimes, you have to ignore test results and just follow your instincts.

THE GREAT WIT OSCAR WILDE once called proctology "without a doubt, the greatest scientific journey mankind has ever embarked upon." A classic Wildean bon mot, overstated for effect. It's an uncomfortable journey, one many doctors are happy to avoid taking, and many patients are equally happy to have them avoid. But it can literally mean the difference between life and death.

Not long ago, George, a retired 88-year-old businessman, came to see me. He was in rough shape. For six months, he'd been suffering from incontinence, diarrhea and weight loss and, while he had seen several doctors, no one seemed able to figure out what was going on, and thus how to help him.

I took a full history. The most significant medical event was that, 12 years earlier, George had fought a bout of prostate cancer and been treated with radiation. Since then, he'd had regular checkups with his urologist at another hospital, including one only four months before I saw him.

"So what kind of investigation was done following your last visit?" I asked him.

"Nothing," George said.

"I can't believe that," I said. "You've had this condition for months."

"Nothing," he insisted. "I can't go anywhere because of the diarrhea."

"Well, what treatment have you been getting?"

"My family doctor gave me cholestyramine. They said I had gallstones."

I knew cholestyramine to be a drug used to remove bile acids from the system. It also causes constipation.

"So how was that diagnosis made?" I asked.

"I don't know," he said.

"Did you have a colonoscopy?"

"No."

I found that very strange, definitely an omission. We then proceeded to do the physical examination, including a rectal probe. There was clear evidence of a rectal mass that could be felt with the fingers. It was blocking the rectum. A CT scan later confirmed its presence. Had it been caught sooner — and it would have been recognized by the simple rectal exam — cancer therapies might have been effective. Unfortunately, this malignancy was too far advanced for chemotherapy or radiation. The only hope was to perform a diverting colostomy, a surgical procedure that allows stool to bypass the blockage caused by the tumour.

We still have our fingers crossed for George's recovery. In the meantime, his quality of life improved dramatically, following the removal of the obstruction by the colostomy.

SOME YEARS AGO, I WAS privileged to work with the young David Naylor, a remarkable epidemiologist who went on to found the Institute for Clinical Evaluative Sciences, housed on the Sunnybrook Hospital campus. Later, he became dean of medicine at the University of Toronto, and later still president of the university. A major proponent of evidence-based medicine, Naylor nonetheless acknowledges its limits, particularly in respect of the large area of medicine known as the Grey Zone.

As Naylor wrote in a 1995 piece in the *Lancet*, in an "era of chronic and expensive disease, there are no vaccines yet for atherosclerosis, cancer, arthritis or AIDS. Until . . . molecular biology pays more concrete dividends we shall be muddling along with what Lewis Thomas characterized as 'halfway technologies.'" Clinical medicine, Naylor wrote, "seems to consist of a few things we know, a few things we think we know (but probably don't) and lots of things we don't know at all."

It is precisely within this large Grey Zone that many physicians must practise. Too often, there is no clear path to diagnosis and treatment. Every step, every decision, is an exercise in uncertainty. An aggressive approach to medical tests might well provide the answer we are seeking. But it also might confuse the issue, providing information that will take us in new and ultimately futile directions. As Naylor says, paraphrasing the great Sir William Osler, "Good clinical medicine will always blend the art of uncertainty with the science of probability."

One patient of mine — Claude, a 40-year-old man from Quebec — provides a case in point. He had been previously diagnosed with inflammatory bowel disease and, while it was under control, other problems developed, including a swelling under his lower jaw. A biopsy uncovered fibrous, non-cancerous tissue, but he was also losing weight and was slightly anemic.

Then, a new complication arose — severe abdominal pain. His family doctor said it was a hernia and sent him to Toronto's Shouldice Hospital for surgical repair. But after they opened him up, they discovered that instead of a hernia, Claude had a large swelling in his lower abdomen. No wonder he was in such pain. His hemoglobin count was down to 100 (the norm is about 120). My own exam confirmed a tender, football-sized mass in his lower abdomen.

But was this cancer or part of a systemic inflammation his body was experiencing? Cancer would take us in one treatment direction, inflammation in another. For several reasons, including an erythrocyte sedimentation rate (ESR) level of 150 and a slightly elevated C-reactive protein count — indices of serious inflammation — we decided to set up a therapeutic trial.

Most such trials, of course, involve hundreds if not thousands of patients. Any verdict about efficacy is based on the results that affect a significant statistical sample. We did not have that luxury. Our sample was one, Claude — thus giving rise to the phrase an "n of 1" trial. The drug we chose was prednisone, a corticosteroid proven over the past six decades to successfully reduce inflammation, though not without some pernicious side effects, including suppression of the body's immune system.

If we were on the right track, then Claude's high ESR and C-reactive numbers would drop, his mass would shrink, his pain would disappear or substantially abate and his hemoglobin would rise.

We started with a large daily dose of prednisone — 60 milligrams — and added methotrexate to curb the steroidal side effects. In two weeks, the fibrous mass had shrunk to the size of a baseball. In six weeks, all our benchmarks for success had been met — general well-being, weight gain, higher hemoglobin count, dramatically reduced mass size and much lower numbers for ESR and C-reactive protein. Over the course of a year, Claude made a complete recovery.

MOST PHYSICIANS, I'D LIKE TO think, are naturally empathetic. It is one of the principal characteristics that motivate many of us to choose medicine in the first place — the instinctive compassion we feel for those who are burdened with disease, and the desire to help them improve or at least come to terms with their illness.

At times, given the weight of caseloads and other demands on our time, the empathy factor can fade to the margins. In fact, there is research to suggest that medical students become less empathetic as they move through the system, a consequence, perhaps, of the growing pressures they face.

And yet for many patients, a display of empathy is what they most need — evidence that their attending doctor cares deeply about their condition and their well-being. One potent supplement to empathy is advocacy, becoming the patient's champion and using resources available to facilitate access to specialists, medical tests, drugs, other therapies and insurance. All these are time-consuming activities, to be sure, but a vital part of the art of medicine.

Kham V., a Canadian originally from Laos, worked as a chef in a Japanese restaurant when, at about the age of 33, he developed Behçet's disease. A rare disorder (named after Turkish dermatologist Hulusi Behçet, who first described it in the 1920s), it inflames the body's blood vessels. For Kham, the first signs of it were painful mouth sores. He was successfully treated for that but, a decade later, developed blood clots in his legs.

He was anti-coagulated with Coumadin, and he recovered, but the clots reappeared on two other occasions, over a period of three months. In fact, they developed despite a very high dosage level of the drug. So we switched to blood-thinning therapies, moving to heparin, which must be administered daily by injection, subcutaneously.

On a chef's modest salary, Kham was not prepared financially to absorb the $12,000 per year cost of the drug. Indeed, to economize, he started to cut back on his injections, first to three times a week, then to once a week. Very quickly, he developed a large, vasculitic leg ulcer — so large, in fact, that the surgeon suggested he might have to sever part of his limb, in order to save him. Fortunately, that wasn't necessary. We quickly returned Kham to his regimen and he slowly recovered.

But the ongoing financial burden was onerous. At that point, I consulted with my chief resident and we agreed to approach the French drug manufacturer, Sanofi-Aventis, and ask them to make a significant donation. Every three months — for the past 12 years — I write a letter requesting a refill, and every three months it arrives in the mail.

The quid pro quo is that we invited Kham to donate his

services to medical education. We have used his case extensively in teaching medical students and residents. Making dozens of trips to the hospital, Kham has allowed himself to be interviewed and examined, to demonstrate the clinical features of recurrent deep-vein thrombosis and life-threatening vasculitic ulcer.

No less important, we make a point of asking students to physically present the three-month supply of heparin to Kham — so that they better appreciate the importance of empathy and the benefits of advocacy.

THE SKILLS INVOLVED IN PRACTISING the art of medicine are not always about diagnosis. Just as often, they pertain to care management, the ability to help your patient live with a condition that may be chronic and incurable, and to ensure they follow the optimum regimen of diet, exercise (where possible) and medication. In others, the core principle is the ancient edict — do no harm. In that context, I'm going to let one of those patients tell the story himself and give him the last word.

A PATIENT'S TESTIMONY — *Brian F.* ————————————

At the age of 55, I developed a dull but persistent pain in my abdomen. My family doctor quickly arranged an ultrasound test, which turned up evidence of abnormality in the area — specifically, fluid buildup. Some weeks went by and the pain disappeared but, for safety's sake, the GP commissioned a second ultrasound. It confirmed the original finding and, because incongruous fluid is seldom a good omen, ordered a CT scan, just to get a better look.

The better look showed both the fluid and a thickening of a layer of fat between the abdominal wall and the internal organs. Any such thickening is potentially significant, so yet more tests were ordered, overseen by a colorectal surgeon. All the blood tests were normal, but a second CT scan yielded identical results to the first — and a conviction that further investigation was needed.

The general feeling was that, despite the encouraging blood tests, a combination of fluid accumulation and cell wall thickening was typically indicative of cancer somewhere in the body. Thus, we proceeded to a tissue biopsy, conducted laparoscopically, as well as something known as a fluid aspiration procedure, so that we could see exactly of what the fluid consisted.

The results were largely positive — no evidence of cancer, but a degree of inflammation. I found the whole thing, which went on for some months, unsettling and a little frightening, just because of the uncertainty. The surgeon assured me that whatever I had, it was unlikely to kill me, but he was concerned enough to refer me to Dr. Ho Ping Kong, or HPK as we call him, whom he said was the smartest man he'd ever met. "Like House — the TV internist," he said, "but much nicer."

Years earlier, the surgeon had been a student of HPK's.

My first visit with Dr. Ho Ping Kong was qualitatively different than any I had had before with any other doctor. He took a lot of time talking to me, asking not only about my symptoms and the history of those symptoms, but about my background, my education, my work, my lifestyle. He was in no hurry to see the next patient and, while I was answering his questions, I could feel him assessing me, observing me. He just takes time and asks a lot of questions that appear to be not medical. Perhaps the oddest question he asked me was whether I still had sex with my wife, although he began by asking if we still slept in the same bedroom. His approach was just more holistic.

He ordered more blood work and, a year later, another set of scans, just to see what if anything had changed. Nothing had. I felt healthy, experienced no pain, had no other medical conditions — no diabetes, no high blood pressure — and was on no medications. Except for the inflammation, I was disgustingly healthy. So HPK just monitored the situation.

I would see him every three or four months or so and occasionally I'd be brought in as a case study when he lectured to students — a case study in how to deal with patients who have some clinical condition, but no known explanation of the origin or cause. Because one of the hardest things to accept — as a patient going through the system — is that we have all these shiny machines and tests that can be done. But the reality is there is still a great deal the medical profession doesn't know and can't explain. So how do you deal with a patient when you don't have an answer? What is the balance between speculation — it could be this and it could be that — and creating a lot of needless anxiety for the patient? My family doctor was reticent because he said, "While we can do the tests, we don't necessarily understand the implications of what we find. We can find things, but is it clinically significant?"

I still have some degree of abnormality and inflammation, but it isn't causing a problem. The tests are looking for changes. If I were lecturing students, I'd say that in order to be a doctor, you need a lot of knowledge of technology, scientific information and the implications of all the numbers. As the knowledge becomes more complex, assimilating it all becomes harder. It is daunting. But at some point you have to focus on the patient as a person, and that's much harder to learn.

It's easy to lose sight of the fact that you are dealing with real people — not a cancer patient, but Joe, a man with a wife and children. It's easy to lose track of that fact. They are not a symptom and they not a disease. I don't know what kind of training future doctors get in the non-technical side of the profession. You really have to pay attention to the patient as a person and it's not easy. We need reassurance and advice about what to do, and what the alternatives are. It's easy to focus on the symptoms because doctors are hard-pressed for time. If you only have 10 minutes with a patient, it's easy to lose sight of the human factor. But it's very, very important.

Dr. MICHAEL BAKER

*A specialist in both general internal medicine and hematology,
Dr. Michael Baker served as physician-in-chief of Toronto General
Hospital and Toronto Western Hospital from 1992 until 2010.
Earlier, as a clinician scientist, he conducted groundbreaking
research showing that leukemia may appear to be in remission
when it is not — studies that led to improvements in understanding of the disease and other cancers. He now holds the Rose Family
Chair in Medicine at the University of Toronto and oversees a
practice for ambulatory medicine. For his contributions to leukemia research, he holds membership in the Order of Canada.*

DR. MICHAEL BAKER'S LONG AND distinguished medical career
divides neatly into two distinct phases. In the first, he was a clinician scientist, investigating acute leukemia. Later, he shifted gears
and became a hospital administrator, although he always insisted
on spending two months a year practising general internal medicine, visiting wards and teaching students. Baker calls it "the most
doctorly thing I do."

During those two months, he tries to demonstrate aspects
of the art of medicine to a group of five residents and students
at the bedside. In a typical scenario, Baker will read the patient's
file, "which tells me that he has, let's say, porphyria, a rare nervous system disorder. Then the junior medical student will access
his or her iPhone to read out everything we might need to know
about the disease. And I'll say, 'Thank you for educating us, but
let's go into the room.' Then I'll demonstrate to these 23-year-old
students what the art of medicine is partly about. I'll go to the
bedside and find a chair and sit so I'm at eye level with the patient,

because to stand in the doorway or to stand towering over the patient suggests detachment and is denigrating."

Then, before he addresses medical issues, Baker seeks to make a human connection with the patient. "I'll look at where they live and discuss local geography. Or if they have an ethnic name and might be an immigrant, I'll ask them where they grew up. And then I'll ask, 'So what brought you to the hospital,' even though I already know the answer. And the answer often has nothing directly to do with whatever is bothering them physically. It may be that she fears she'll be too sick to make it to her son's wedding on Sunday. So that is my contribution to the art of medicine for students who think it's all about what you learn on your iPhone."

Baker says he adopted that practice long before the era of the internet. "Before that, I did it in resentment of everyone constantly looking at the patient's chart. The point is to use the knowledge base you have to help the patient in front of you."

Of course, the challenge is larger than that. There's a good chance, Baker notes, that the patient is suffering not only from porphyria, but from diabetes, heart failure and asthma. "So there are 28 things one could possibly do. It's like trying to discuss the influence of the history of the United States on its relationship with Europe. Where do you start? How do you prioritize? That's what a case can feel like. There's a ton of information about the illnesses, the diagnosis, the treatment, so the art form — and it is an art form — is integrating all the facts with the human factor: her fear of missing the son's wedding, the fact that she's scared to death and is the caregiver for a husband who has dementia."

Baker says all the medical students are "disgustingly brilliant and multi-talented. But there is no textbook or computer program to model integration and decision making that filters all of this information, the clinical and the personal, the social and the psychological issues." Teaching that, he says, requires a human model.

The rise of medical subspecialization, Baker allows, has created a gap into which many patients have fallen. On the one hand, the availability of a subspecialist with crucial expertise has made a dramatic impact on patient outcomes. "But if you narrow your focus, you lose the broad picture," he says.

The system's solution has been to make the family doctor the patient's quarterback, integrating and coordinating all the relevant tests, information and treatments. "But there is so much technical expertise that the family doctor is easily overwhelmed for understandable reasons. There's no way they can keep up. So the gap between the family doctors, as good and knowledgeable and compassionate as they are, and our specialized hospital is too wide."

There are several ways to bridge the gap, he suggests. One is ambulatory clinic groups, which Baker calls a rudimentary but essentially good idea. Another is the expansion of family clinics to include nurses, nurse practitioners, social workers and pharmacists — making a wider knowledge base accessible to patients.

"But what I personally support is what Herbert Ho Ping Kong is doing at his Centre for Excellence in Education and Practice, which is to embed a sophisticated general internist in an outpatient clinic setting. And it then becomes the internist's job to navigate and coordinate complex patient care — patients, for example, with multi-system disease."

In this model, the patient is given the internist's email address and personal cell phone number. For routine matters, the patient can call the secretary and arrange to speak to the doctor. But for urgent matters, they can access the doctor directly and get a response the same day. "And if the patient thinks he is so sick that he needs to go to the emergency room," Baker says, "he calls me first, because I know him and I'll know whether it can wait. Or if he really needs to go there, I can call the ER and ensure that he is seen promptly and instruct them what to do."

Baker now runs exactly that type of practice from his Toronto General Hospital offices. "I maybe get a private phone call once every three weeks. It takes me less than five minutes." Once, Baker was in New York for a weekend when a patient called. He was running a fever of 38.5 degrees Celsius, but was reluctant to go to the emergency room. "I insisted he go immediately. Knowing the patient and knowing he was immune deficient, a 38-degree fever is the tipping point. He needed antibiotics. So I sent him to the ER, he was admitted for a week, and he was fine."

Recently, Baker received an email from a patient concerned about a nodule discovered on his prostate gland. He already had an elevated PSA — the prostate specific antigen marker in the blood, often seen as a precursor of cancer. "So what does he do? His GP discovers the nodule and says, 'You need to see a urologist.' That will take three months, minimum. The GP writes the reference letter, but the urologist receives a thousand of these letters every month and doesn't know which case is more urgent. But if I see the patient, I can then call a urologist colleague and arrange a quick consultation. So that, too, is the art of medicine — general internist playing a role, calming the fears of a worried man."

For that system to work more broadly, thousands of new internists would be needed. "So it's not *the* solution, but *a* solution."

It's a solution that could also apply to patients suffering from Grey Zone illnesses — pain, fatigue, low-grade fever and debilitation. "Family doctors will tell you that their most common presenting problem is fatigue. Dealing with that is for sure an art form, because you have to determine if it's a serious, recognized illness, like lupus or arthritis, or something more esoteric or something psychological. We currently rely on family doctors to sort this out, but it tends to require another sophisticated opinion." Even then specialists, Baker says, are likely to identify not what the ailment is, but what it isn't — "this isn't lupus" or "it isn't a stroke." "And that brings it back to the GP, who may not be equipped to do a proper evaluation. So again, a general internist can be helpful here in assimilating all the facts and using technology wisely to come to a diagnosis."

It is critical, Baker says, not only to know when to order, for example, an MRI or a CT scan, but how to read them — "to filter out the signals from the noise." Many such scans will turn up ambiguous dots — possible growths on lungs, liver, kidneys or stomach, which may be malignant or benign.

"The patient may request these tests, but you can't indiscriminately order them," Baker says. "And explaining why they may not be a good idea takes confidence, and the application of the art of medicine. There is such a thing as too much information, which may do more harm than good."

A busy family doctor facing 10 patients an hour can be forgiven for needing hard information and ordering them, he adds. And some physicians practise legal medicine: fearing malpractice suits, they reflexively cover themselves by ordering tests. "But a good, sophisticated internist will be cautious."

CHAPTER 2

STARTING OUT

The whole art of medicine is in observation . . . but to educate the eye to see, the ear to hear and the finger to feel takes time, and to make a beginning, to start a man on the right path, is all that you can do.
— Sir William Osler

I ALWAYS KNEW THAT I would become a doctor.

I knew it not, as one might expect, because my parents coaxed me toward the profession, but because of my childhood nanny. Let me explain.

I was the third child born — in 1939 — into a family of 10 in Summerfield, a country town in the district of Clarendon, some distance from the Jamaican capital of Kingston. My parents were both Hakka Chinese, a minority that, through the centuries, has exerted enormous influence in China's political and social history.

My grandfather had arrived a generation earlier from China to work in the Caribbean cane sugar fields as an indentured labourer — one unglorified step up from slave. In time, some 10,000 Chinese would settle in Jamaica and, through thrift and hard work, become prosperous, particularly in the retail trade.

So prosperous, in fact, that by the mid-1960s, racial tensions with the indigenous Jamaican community were bubbling up.

From cane — the world's largest food crop and a staple of the Jamaican economy, then and now — was derived sucrose, which was used to make chocolate, molasses, rum and several other products. At one time, cane sugar was considered so valuable that empires would literally barter away valuable territories for it. It was in exchange for the sugar-cane-rich fields of Surinam, for example, that the Dutch ceded New Netherlands — New York — to the British in 1674. A century later, ending the Seven Years' War, France ceded what it called "a few acres of snow" — namely, Canada — to the English, in return for the cane plantations of Guadeloupe, Martinique and St. Lucia.

At the age of 16, my father, Percy Ho Ping Kong, came from Canton in the mid-1930s, fleeing hunger in China. He became an assistant in a Chinese-owned grocery shop. Somehow, without going to school, he managed to learn to read and write grammatically correct English. A thrifty man, he later saved enough funds to buy and successfully run his own grocery shop for many years.

My mother, Mary, arrived four years later, having been betrothed to him at the age of 12. She was also very smart — at once resourceful and creative. She knew instinctively how to build and fix things. In fact, after we moved to Kingston, my parents decided to build a house. For some reason, the hired contractor was unable to complete the job, so my mother took over and organized the entire project. We grew our own vegetables and raised ducks and chickens in the backyard. From the products of that garden and farmhouse, my mother made the most delicious meals. Her food was so good and so locally renowned, that it wasn't uncommon for restaurant owners to stop by for a small discussion about recipes. And she had healing hands: once, one of our ducks became sick, unable to move, and my mother asked me — I must have been about 10 years old — to hold it still while she performed surgery. She took a razor blade and made a careful incision in the neck. I can't say definitively whether this procedure was curative, but the next day, the bird got up and walked.

We were not rich, but almost every family with children in Jamaica was able to afford a nanny. Ours was a young Jamaican woman named Mum Robinson. One day when I was five — I remember it vividly — she told my brother Lloyd that he would become a lawyer (which he did not) and that I would become a doctor.

It was not a game — she was deadly serious. Although uneducated, she knew that the professions were important. We all had heard about a certain Dr. Robb, a distinguished physician/surgeon who lived in our district. People came from all over the country to see him. I was to be like him, she said. After that, I never thought about it again. I knew what I would become and never deviated from the path.

My parents' marriage was largely happy, but my father definitely came from the old school of Chinese thinking, in which men were dominant and women were subservient. He was prepared to work hard, and he did, but he expected to be served at mealtimes and would frequently complain, usually in the direction of my mother, if he perceived something wrong. I found this increasingly hard to endure as, I'm sure, did my mother.

One day, when I was 12, he came in for dinner and set off on one of his typical rants. I was cutting cod fish in the same room and I suddenly turned to him, still chopping, and shouted, "Poppa! Enough. That's it!" I'm sure it was a shock to see his son rebuke him like that.

But he got the message. He shut up, not just at that moment, but forever after. As far as I know, he never said another unkind word to or about my mother. The incident also revealed something about me — that I could be tough when I needed to be.

For some reason, my formal education did not start until the age of seven. It began in the Jamaican equivalent of a one-room schoolhouse, with a single teacher and students that ranged in age from seven to 16. But I was very fortunate — I befriended a young Lebanese boy named Bobby Abisted, about 13. He became my tutor and really helped me prepare for high school. He taught me how to read quickly and more critically, how to teach myself, a skill for which I remain in his debt to this day.

I attended high school at St. George's, a Jesuit institution in Kingston, founded in 1850 by 21 Spanish Jesuits exiled from Colombia during a period of religious persecution.

On my first day, the school conducted its usual outdoor assembly and roll call — 1,000 students aged 12–19. They called 999 names, every one except mine. I stood alone in the square, dressed in short pants.

The headmaster, Father Charles McMullen, approached me.

"Well," he said, in his thick Boston accent. "And who are you?"

"I am Herbert Ho, sir."

He peered down at his list. "There's no Herbert Ho here."

"Don't you remember, sir? I saw you last week. I paid my fees."

"What's your father's name?"

"His name is Ho Ping Kong," I said.

"Son, your name is too short," he declared. "From now on, you will be Herbert Ho Ping Kong."

Thus was my name changed — on the spot. And thus did it remain. It was probably a good thing. There are literally thousands of people named Herbert Ho in the world, but very few named Herbert Ho Ping Kong.

Because of Bobby Abisted's tutoring, I managed to complete two years in one during my first year at St. George's. My favourite course was biology, largely because my teacher, Father Hennessy, would often engage us in more popular discussions, including girls — a rather unorthodox topic in a Jesuit school — or social issues such as slavery.

The school's teaching standards were set high. Virtually all of the teachers had earned master's degrees or the equivalent. Thus, in effect, we received university standard teaching in physics, chemistry, biology and other courses.

The Jesuits believed in educating the whole person. Thus, in addition to academic performance, they stressed such things as speaking skills and athletics. I played many sports, but truthfully excelled at none of them. In the end, I was described as the school's shortest high jumper, its slowest sprinter and its slowest pace bowler in cricket. But I did captain one of the cricket teams and was named head boy of the school in my final year. Although I represented a racial minority, it wasn't unusual for a Chinese youth to win such distinction. The Jesuits saw everyone as equal and treated everyone as equal, without having to preach about it.

As head boy, I was also expected to demonstrate leadership qualities. One day, we were having an elocution lesson with the same Father McMullen. A friend, Richard Chin, was called on to speak to the class, but suddenly froze. He did not recall the assignment and was unprepared for the occasion. In retrospect, it might have been my fault for neglecting to give him the assignment. In any event, I decided to come to his assistance.

"I think I'm the one who is supposed to give the speech," I lied.

"Alright," said McMullen. "And what are you going to speak about?"

"The Yangtze River in China, sir."

And with that, I launched into an extemporaneous 15-minute speech on a subject I knew almost nothing about. I described the river's considerable length and the chromatic origins of its name, and the plant and animal life that lived along its shores.

Afterward, Father McMullen said, "You did well, Ho Ping Kong, but you must learn to pronounce your 'th' sounds better."

As I approached the end of my high school years, I went to see McMullen to discuss where I might go to university. Most of my friends were headed to the United States. And my older sister, Joyce, had earlier won a scholarship to study in Indiana.

He said, "You are not going abroad. You're staying here at the University of the West Indies to study medicine. If you go to America, you'll do four years of liberal arts and then apply to medicine. But you are smart enough to go straight into medicine here. It's a more direct route."

There was no further discussion.

And that's exactly what I did. In 1959, I entered a six-year program that began with basic science and led to a degree in medicine. The class numbered 29 students. We shared a campus residence with older students who became our mentors. I particularly remember a fourth-year student, Hornet Seawar from Guyana, always immaculately dressed in a white hospital coat. His behaviour was likewise exemplary. They taught not only how to dress, but to always act professionally and to never miss a call. Like the Jesuits, they taught us as much by example as by words.

ONE OF MY SEMINAL, CAREER-FORMING experiences took place in the emergency ward at University Hospital of the West Indies in Kingston in 1968. The ER department was a busy place, seeing 40 to 60 patients a day, although most of what we saw and treated was not medically complex. One day, I was asked to see a 21-year-old man who'd been shot by police, while he was fleeing a robbery attempt. The report said he had an abscess on the back of his right leg, at the entry site of the bullet wound. My assignment was to make an incision and drain it.

Examining the leg, I noticed that it was red, hot, tender and pulsating, an indication to me that the patient had developed what is known as a popliteal aneurysm. I could hear the leakage of the artery when I put the stethoscope on it. Fortunately, I did not use a scalpel to drain the presumed abscess. Instead, I used my eyes and ears to diagnose what was really happening.

It was perhaps my first powerful object lesson in the importance of not always relying on the evidence already assembled — and using my hands, eyes and ears to make the diagnosis. Nowadays, the aneurysm would likely be detected with ultrasound scanners but, as this case indicates, such tools, while important, aren't essential if a primary care physician uses the basic human skill set of his senses.

Sometimes, the correct answers can be found just by knowing how to ask the right questions. I recall another case from those early years of residency — a young man who presented with severe abdominal pain and a history of a gastric ulcer. The general concern was that the ulcer might be perforating. After posing a set of questions, I learned that he was diabetic, but had not taken his insulin for three days. He was badly dehydrated and hyperventilating. I was pretty sure I knew what the trouble was — diabetic ketoacidosis, which, in its acute stages, can give you severe abdominal pain. Undiagnosed, dehydration sets in and blood volume declines, complicated by severe electrolyte imbalance. Untreated, it is potentially lethal. So understanding a patient's history is vitally important.

Not long after, I was to confront another case that would change my life forever. The late American physician Walsh McDermott, who edited the textbook that became the bible for many internists (*Cecil Textbook of General Medicine*), used to say that the best doctors were allowed to make no more than five serious mistakes in their career. I was about to make my first.

A young man of 27 arrived in the emergency department complaining of headache and a slight weakness on his right side. Our initial diagnosis, based on a lumbar puncture, was encephalitis, an inflammation likely caused by a virus infecting the lining of brain. His blood-sugar ratios seemed to support this hypothesis. The mistake I made was in not paying sufficient attention to the so-called localizing signs — in this case, his right-side weakness. That should have suggested something other than encephalitis, probably a space-occupying lesion.

I was at the end of my shift and went home for 12 hours. But the case stayed with me and, the more I thought about it, the more certain I became that something else was going on. When

THE ART OF MEDICINE

I returned to the hospital the next morning, I promptly ordered a carotid angiogram. It turned up evidence of a cerebral abscess. We immediately tried to drain it, but we were too late. The young man died. Had I not waited those critical 12 hours, he might have been saved. We should have done the angiogram right away.

My mistake haunted me. The condition was something I was aware of and should have detected, but I'd been misled by the test results. Had I bothered to discuss the case with colleagues, they might have reminded me to consider other possibilities. Since then, and to this day, I make it a practice to confer with other physicians, even students, on difficult cases, because you never know where a good idea might come from. It's always helpful to talk about the case. The sorrow of that unnecessary death lingered with me for months.

Two weeks later, just as my shift was ending, I heard a commotion coming from the nursing station of the main ER ward. A patient, already admitted for headaches, suddenly appeared to go crazy. He'd left his hospital room, leapt on top of the nurses' station and begun to urinate. I heard people screaming, "Call the police!"

I approached him carefully.

"Sam," I said, "are you still having the headaches?"

"Yes, doctor, really bad headaches, like I told you before."

"Well, come down and go back to your bed and I'll look after you."

So he climbed down and went back to his room. I thought the erratic behaviour might be evidence of a brain abscess on his frontal lobe — thus the lack of inhibition demonstrated on the nurses' desk. I promptly ordered a brain angiogram, which confirmed my diagnosis. We rushed him into neurosurgery to drain his abscess and managed to save his life.

Would I have made the same decision if, just two weeks earlier, I hadn't failed to consider the possibility of an abscess and had lost that patient? I'd like to think so. But there's no doubt the proximity of the two cases made me more alert to the possibility of abscess. In any event, it provided a valuable lesson for me: even when you make a mistake, you can't allow it to affect your performance. Feel regret, certainly— but don't get too down, because you can access the experience, like an archive, in future cases, and learn from it.

I was able to do just that with two patients I treated some 40 years apart. The first was a Jamaican woman who presented with a swollen abdomen and a distended vein in her neck. Chest x-rays later provided the diagnosis: constrictive pericarditis, the calcification of the pericardium, the double-layered membrane that surrounds the heart. Her condition — very rare — was likely the legacy of a previous bout of tuberculosis, but it had persisted for so long that, by the time we saw her, nothing remedial could be done. That was 1966.

Four decades later, a colleague at Toronto's Mount Sinai Hospital asked me to examine Edna, a 29-year-old young mother of three, who was complaining of fatigue, shortness of breath and a stomach swollen with seemingly inexplicable fluid buildup (ascites). There was no peripheral edema (leg or ankle swelling); this was an important consideration because, if her legs had been swollen, it might have suggested right-sided heart failure. But there was a history of rheumatoid arthritis.

Edna had been to see both a respirologist and a cardiologist, and made several trips to the emergency ward, with no diagnosis and no relief. But almost as soon as I saw her, I knew what the problem was — constrictive pericarditis. Despite the rareness of the condition, or perhaps because of it, the telltale sign was immediately apparent. She had the same distended neck vein (known as a jugular venous distension) and ascites (an accumulation of fluid in the peritoneal cavity) that I had seen years earlier in Jamaica, but without peripheral edema. I had not seen it since.

"Don't worry," I told her. "I know what's wrong with you. We can treat you."

A cardiac MRI verified the diagnosis and indicated that the pericardium was four millimetres thick, instead of what it should have been — one millimetre. Using a relatively simple but tedious surgical procedure, the calcified "wallpaper" around the membrane was removed — pericardial stripping. Within three weeks, she was back to normal. Fortunately, she has been trouble-free since then.

I WAS SOMETIMES, THOUGH NOT always, the top student in medical school, but I worked hard and earned respectable grades. In addition to the formal academic program, I routinely spent another 30 hours a week studying and reading journals and related material. If I only spent 20 hours at these activities, I felt guilty. My only real "downtime" was Sunday mornings, when I listened to classical music on the radio and read the newspapers.

Hard work paid off in the end, as I earned the gold medal in medicine at graduation. At the time I was close friends with Robin Sahoy, a Guyanese student who became a surgeon. He spent many long hours, as I did, trying to memorize parts of *Gray's Anatomy*, the classic medical text. One day, he made me a bet: that he could stay awake longer than I could. I took the bet. I was 22 years old and, as young men often do, thought I was invincible. We had a biochemistry exam scheduled for seven nights hence. I stayed up the entire time; he succumbed to sleep after six nights. I earned an A plus; Robin got an A minus.

I haven't done anything quite so foolish since then. But the experience did show me that, thereafter, being on call for 24 or 48 hours would never be a problem.

I studied under many brilliant physicians in Jamaica. One of them was Dr. Donald Gore, an upper-crust Jamaican surgeon who had worked at the Columbia University–affiliated New York Presbyterian Hospital and then returned home to practise. He had great technical skills in the operating room, as well as unerring judgment but, to the chagrin of many of us, a very short fuse as a teacher. That veneer of toughness, of course, is considered part of the makeup of surgeons generally, but in my experience, the stereotype was wrong. Most of them were gentle souls; Gore was the exception.

I worked with him for three months. On ward rounds, he would demand that we succinctly summarize a patient's case in no more than three sentences.

He'd typically say to one student, "Okay, describe the case."

"This is a 25-year-old man admitted yesterday with abdominal pain and a fever."

"Three sentences, doctor. Three sentences."

"His pain was crampy and he had vomiting."

"One sentence to go, doctor."

"His mucous membranes were pink."

"That's three. Diagnosis?"

Then, he'd cut the student off and we'd be left hanging, with no diagnosis. Then he'd do the same thing with another student doctor, and then another. No one seemed able to distill the essence of the case into three sentences.

"Sorry, guys," he'd say. "You obviously don't know the cases. We are finished teaching for this week. When I say three sentences, I mean three sentences."

The next week, it was my turn.

"Okay, Ho Ping Kong, what have got for me?"

"Sir, this is a 35-year-old man who presented with weight loss, tachycardia, a pulse rate of 140 per minutes. He has Stellwag's sign [an indication of Graves' hyperthyroidism in the eyes] and I believe he has Graves' disease. We need to operate on him after we control it."

Onerous as his challenge was, we all eventually learned to synopsize the essence of the case in three sentences.

ALTHOUGH TECHNOLOGICALLY MEDICINE in Jamaica often lagged behind other parts of the developed world, our clinical care was on par. That was largely owing to the presence of such giants as Dr. Eric Cruickshank, a former prisoner of war who taught us internal medicine and neurology, and Dr. Ronnie Irving, a British-trained Jamaican who may be the most astute physician I ever saw. Irving had extraordinary powers of intuition; he could diagnose you simply by sitting at your bedside.

In terms of a specialty, my first choice was nephrology. My mentor, Dr. George Alleyne, had studied the same field in Boston with a group that would ultimately make major advances in our understanding of the body's acid-based balances — William B. Schwartz and Arnold S. Relman. Alleyne invited me to spend a year doing research at his Tropical Metabolic Research Unit in Kingston, and I agreed, launching a project to examine renal malfunction in sickle-cell anemia, an often fatal genetic blood disorder common in the West Indies.

With sickle-cell anemia, patients experience acutely painful crises — ischemia and/or infarction of the lungs, bone and other internal organs. The prevailing theory was that the pain was caused by acidosis. In healthy people, the acid would be eliminated in the urine. The hypothesis was that sickle-cell anemics carried a defect in urinary acidification, and thus had trouble excreting an acid load.

In my first experiment, we administered ammonium chloride, a recognized method of testing the kidneys' ability to deal with acid loads. Our studies confirmed the defect. I owe my Ph.D. to that research project, which was supervised by Dr. George Alleyne and ultimately published in the *Lancet*.

The theory, however, wasn't entirely accurate. My patients were not as acidotic as we expected. In fact, their general pH levels were significantly higher than what the medical literature suggested — largely because the hyperventilation associated with the disease and pain yielded what is known as respiratory alkalosis. Our second paper, recording these additional observations, thus changed basic views of physiology: acidosis was not always the cause of painful crises for sickle-cell patients.

But I was not destined to become a bench researcher. What I really wanted to be was a clinician and a teacher.

In 1970, to continue my studies in nephrology, I went to Britain on a Commonwealth Scholarship. Dialysis, as a medical treatment, was still in its infancy, but we had been the first to deploy peritoneal dialysis for leptospirosis, a bacterial infection that causes kidney dysfunction and can be fatal. After a few months in London at St. Thomas' Hospital, I planned to join the new dialysis unit at the Royal Infirmary of Edinburgh to complete my training in internal medicine and nephrology; after nine months, I would become a specialist in nephrology.

It was not to be. Not long before I was scheduled to leave London, a colleague in Edinburgh called to report that, in a matter of a few weeks, four staff members — doctors and nurses — attached to the dialysis unit had died from acute liver failure. Fulminant hepatitis, a lethal swelling of the liver, was suspected, although, at the time, we did not clearly understand that hepatitis manifests itself in different forms, A, B and C. We now know that this outbreak was caused by hepatitis B.

I was immediately told that, unless I had no previous exposure to hepatitis, I would not be allowed to join the group. As it happened, I'd had such exposure. When I was 16, I'd attended a summer camp in Jamaica, which used septic toilets. I became jaundiced — I could not swallow my saliva, it was so nausea-inducing — and was soon diagnosed with hepatitis. The sight, taste, even the thought of food made me want to vomit. There was no treatment, but the presiding physician assured me I would not die. I had contracted hepatitis — as we later discovered, the milder A version.

My history with the disease would have prevented me from gaining entry to the unit, although I likely would have made the same decision on my own. I would be in England with my wife, our three children and my mother-in-law and would not have wanted to expose them to whatever germs I might have picked up in the Royal Infirmary of Edinburgh.

I was naturally disappointed but, having been trained as a general internist, I was able to shift course and join Edinburgh's Western General Hospital to hone my skills in general medicine. I was, by this time, more than a little cocky about my talents — in fact, too cocky. I'd been a top student, had published research in the best medical journals and earned my Ph.D. in physiology. But I was about to earn my comeuppance.

To earn my MRCP — a diploma of Membership of the Royal Colleges of Physicians of the United Kingdom — I had to pass two exams. Two weeks after arriving in London I breezed through the multiple-choice segment without any problem. Moving from London to Edinburgh I encountered Dr. Batty, my stately, imperious Scottish examiner for two case studies involving live patients.

"Dr. Ho, where are you from?" he began.

"Kingston, Jamaica, sir."

"Ah . . . A great place . . . And how long have you been here, Dr. Ho?"

"Two weeks, sir, in Edinburgh."

"Hmmm," he said. "Not long enough."

We were not off to an auspicious start. The patient presented to me was a 50-year-old woman. I began by examining her spleen and found it massively enlarged — I'd seen about 50 similar cases in Jamaica — and was, as usual, confident about my diagnosis.

After no more than 15 seconds, I said, "Sir, this woman has a massive splenomegaly [a very big spleen]. There are only four things that could cause it. In Africa or Malaysia, it could be kala azar or malaria. But in Scotland, it's either going to be myelofibrosis or chronic myeloid leukemia."

Dr. Batty turned to me. "I did note that you had not been here long enough."

I said, "Sir, if you show me the patient's blood slide, I will confirm the diagnosis."

So he passed me the slide and the problem was indeed transparent. "Sir, the slide clearly shows a leukoerythroblastic picture [a combination of abnormal red and white blood cells]. This patient has myelofibrosis." It had taken me 30 seconds.

He said, "Doctor, you have not been here long enough."

As a result, he failed me — the first and last time I failed an exam in my life. I was devastated and deeply despondent.

My wife and our three children and I lived in an apartment overlooking Edinburgh's Holyrood Park, within sight of the city's famous Holyrood Palace. We often went for walks on its grounds. The park called itself home to 1,000 sheep, only one of which was black. After failing the exam, I spent a lot of time looking for that black sheep, which obviously I identified with myself.

Was it racism? I really don't know. Perhaps Dr. Batty genuinely believed that one had to be immersed in British culture and medicine for at least a year before earning the MRCP designation.

The next day I was summoned to an audience with Dr. John Macleod, chairman of the department of medicine at Western General Hospital and editor of a definitive textbook used at the time, *Davidson's Principles and Practice of Medicine*.

He asked me to sit down and said, "On behalf of the Royal College of Physicians, I need to apologize to you, Dr. Ho. You did not really fail the exam. Unfortunately, the mark has been formally entered and we cannot undo it. What we can do, however, is remove Dr. Batty from the examining board, and that has already been done. Moreover, for the duration of your stay here, we'd like to offer you a position as a paid tutor, at a salary of six pounds per week." In 1970 terms, that was a small fortune.

I accepted the position and his comments with gratitude, and my wife promptly went out and bought a set of Royal Doulton china, which we still have 43 years later.

But I still felt badly about what had happened. That failure would change my life, for the better. It made me less egotistical, a little less assured of my opinions. I had modelled my behaviour on brilliant but very no-nonsense physicians I'd known in Jamaica, such as Drs. Cruickshank and Irving. After this, I softened a bit and became a little more tolerant, I'd like to think, of people who failed. Thus, I hope, did many others ultimately benefit from my unfortunate exam experience.

I had my first opportunities to do that almost as soon as I returned to Jamaica, in the fall of 1971. As a newly minted lecturer in medicine, I introduced the country's first coronary care unit (a grand total of two beds); the local Chinese Benevolent Society put up $10,000 for our first machines. I also trained young doctors planning to do medical fellowships in the U.K. on how to prepare for their exams. At least, they would not have to deal with the likes of Dr. Batty.

One day, just before dinner, I received an urgent call at home. A 19-year-old woman — the fiancée of one of my interns — was recovering from surgery for appendicitis, when her heart rate suddenly began to spike to 200 beats per minute, a potentially life-threatening situation. Even with infections, heart rates are seldom faster than 120 to 160 beats per minute. I rushed to the hospital.

Her temperature, when I arrived, was about 105 degrees Fahrenheit. There was no evidence of septicemia, though I doubted whether that condition would induce such a massively elevated heart rate. I did think briefly about malignant hyperthermia, the result of exposure to certain anesthetic drugs.

However, on examination, I observed and felt a swelling in her neck, and listening (with the stethoscope) detected a bruit over the thyroid. I immediately concluded that this was a thyroid storm, an episode of acute hyperthyroidism that, untreated, would certainly take her life. We promptly injected beta blockers to reduce the heart rate and used ice and fans to bring her temperature down, and rehydrate her. It took 12 hours, but she was eventually stabilized and her life was saved.

Some 40 years later, an old Jamaican friend of mine was visiting Greece when, by coincidence, he met this woman and her husband; they had married and subsequently relocated to the United States. I was delighted to learn that after that very close call, she had enjoyed a long and productive life.

MY WORK IN JAMAICA WAS challenging and fulfilling, but at that time the country was undergoing social and political turmoil, precipitated by its socialist leaning and Fidel Castro–admiring prime minister, Michael Manley. I had no objection in principle to the notion of income redistribution that his ruling party championed; the growing problem was that its ideology was accompanied by a campaign of social stigmatization and violence directed at anyone deemed to be part of an economic or intellectual elite. Manley's policies were effectively polarizing the nation.

Years earlier, the venom had been aimed at Jamaica's Hakka Chinese community, which maintained a virtual monopoly on retail trade, owning the vast majority of dry goods shops and supermarkets. A series of riots broke out in 1965, during which eight people died and several Chinese-owned stores were burned to the ground, including, on the evening before my final medical exam, my father's. It was a traumatic experience. He never worked again.

Now, half a decade later, members of the university staff were becoming the targets of renewed violence. The other doctors and I needed police escorts to reach the hospital safely.

One day, I attended an academic lecture that was to be delivered by a prominent visiting professor from Glasgow. We were comfortably seated in the auditorium when a group of protesters burst into the room and declared, "We've come to get the white man," referring to one of my fellow lecturers. The chairman managed to stare them down, but the event crystallized my thinking and ultimately my resolve.

I went home, shed my tears and decided to emigrate. My wife, Barbara, fully supported the decision. "I can't continue to work like this," I told my supervisor.

Thus, in 1972, with a heavy heart, I actively began to explore professional opportunities abroad.

A

PSYCHIATRIST'S

PERSPECTIVE

Dr. DAVID GOLDBLOOM

Born in Montreal, Dr. Goldbloom was raised there and in Halifax. Advised by his father, Richard, to study something other than science "and learn about the rest of the world," even if he eventually intended to practise medicine, Goldbloom took an undergraduate degree at Harvard in government and won a Rhodes Scholarship. At Oxford, he studied physiology, earning an M.A., and then returned to Montreal to study medicine at McGill University. By then, he had married the former Nancy Epstein, an ophthalmologist and daughter of Dr. Nate Epstein, who had been recruited from Montreal to become founding chairman of the psychiatry department at McMaster's medical school. In 1985, after hearing a lecture by the Clarke Institute's director Paul Garfinkel, Goldbloom moved to Toronto, practising first at Toronto General and then becoming chief of staff at the Clarke. When the Centre for Addiction and Mental Health (CAMH) was created in 1998, he was named its physician-in-chief, serving in that position for five years before becoming its senior medical advisor.

IT ISN'T OFTEN THAT YOU encounter a physician who begins a conversation with the statement, "Medicine cures almost nothing." Such is the view, however, of Dr. David Goldbloom, senior medical advisor at the Centre for Addiction and Mental Health in Toronto and professor of psychiatry at the University of Toronto.

For Goldbloom, the art of medicine is about engaging patients in ways that allow doctors to understand, and to offer help and hope. Can hope be offered in every case? "I think it's rare you can't provide them with some kind of hope." But hope, he cautions, does not necessarily mean cure.

"This search for the cure plays into the mythic aspirations of people who are ill," he says. "The daily toil of medicine is rarely about cure. The daily toil of medicine is about helping people live with what they have, facilitate their best possible adaptation to it, minimize the intrusion of their symptoms on their functioning and their quality of life and maintain the hope that things will improve. That is the art of medicine."

Even people who are dying, Goldbloom insists, have hopes — hopes about what the nature of their death will be like. Palliative medicine, he says, has taught the medical community a great deal about hope. The idea that hope is extinguished if the patient is terminal is based on a much too narrow construct — that hope is cure. Goldbloom cites the instructive epithet of 19th-century American sanitarium physician Edward Trudeau: "to cure rarely, to relieve often, to comfort always."

It is understanding, he says, that generates a diagnosis. But diagnosis is only a small part of the art of medicine's complex equation. Diagnosis pinpoints the disease, "but the illness is the context." And diagnosis is based on a two-word principle: pattern recognition. "That is what doctors do, day in and day out," Goldbloom says. And if they couldn't do it, if every patient presented with symptoms that defied pattern recognition, "they'd be terrified," he says.

The art of medicine extends the challenge. It asks physicians to graft that highly reproducible pattern onto the unique pathway that constitutes a human life and context and experience.

It isn't uncommon to find patients who will tell friends and family, "I have a great doctor." But what, Goldbloom asks, do they mean by that? What they typically mean is that "he or she spends time with me. They really listen to what I'm saying. And they know their stuff. Few patients have the ability to evaluate their doctor's medical skills, whether diagnostic or surgical. But they know if they have a good or bad doctor, and that judgment taps directly into the art of medicine."

In one well-known experiment about care, doctors were asked to approach their patient and either stand or sit by the bedside. Both the standing doctors and the sitting doctors stayed in the room for precisely the same length of time. But in every instance, patients perceived doctors who sat as having stayed longer.

Goldbloom maintains that the humane side of medicine can be taught, but "the worst place to teach it is in the classroom." The best place, he suggests, is on rounds, in clinics or in doctors' offices. Medicine, historically, has been an apprenticeship profession, but "there's been some erosion of that concept." In part, it's the result of the explosion of scientific knowledge, which new doctors are expected to absorb and master.

For one year, Goldbloom taught part of a course in the art and science of clinical medicine at the University of Toronto. The mandate involved leading students into the hospital for first time and letting them interview and examine patients. "My first interview took about six hours," Goldbloom recalls of his own student days. "I had to take a dinner break in the middle, and I still left out the abdominal exam."

For his teaching gig, Goldbloom found himself at Toronto Western Hospital's neurosurgical unit. He initially feared that all the patients' ailments would be too similar medically but, while they were, the students were nevertheless exposed to a diverse range of people. He remembers one older Chinese patient who had broken a vertebra in his neck, but had not been paralyzed and was making a good recovery. The student assigned to interview him did a good job. At the end, Goldbloom told the man this was the students' first day in the hospital — did he have any advice to give them about being a good doctor?

"You must love your patients," the old man said. "Here, I see some who do and some who don't."

For Goldbloom, it was an extraordinary moment and he felt privileged to have been part of it as a witness. Months later, he had occasion to bump into several of the students in the room that night, and the elder Chinese gentleman's remarks were "etched like granite" in their memories.

Loving every patient — or even giving them the impression that they are loved — is a tall order, he allows. The demands on a physician's time constitute one limiting factor. But so is the social reality that not all patients are loveable. Part of the challenge of the art of medicine, he suggests, is "finding things to like in people you don't like. Even with a pest, there has to be something you can connect with. You have to work at it because, if you don't, the patient will pick up on your negative attitude. You might be withholding or punitive or avoidant. You might take a holiday when he or she is booked for an appointment."

Doctors therefore require a level of self-awareness, because just as there will be patients they don't like, there will be patients they may like too much. They give them too much time and attention, or stray into ethical boundary violations. Both can impact on their ability to be a good physician.

Not long ago, a colleague of Goldbloom had to deliver a negative medical report to a young woman. The patient had a difficult condition for which there was no known remedy. His colleague agonized over how to deliver the news. He read books by other doctors on that very subject. He sought the opinion of other doctors. And he spent many hours just thinking the issue through, weighing how best to convey the difficult prognosis.

"There is no one single right way to do it," he says, "but there are many bad ways to do it." During his years as a student on a surgical rotation, he watched one presiding resident march in to see a post-operative patient and announce without preamble, "You've got cancer. I'll see you in a while."

"Why did you do that?" an incredulous Goldbloom later asked the resident.

"Because in my experience, after you tell them they have cancer, they don't hear anything else you say anyway. So I let them stew and then go back and talk to them."

Of course, there was a time when it was normative for physicians not to tell patients, particularly the elderly, that they had cancer. A conspiracy of silence would reign. The children would be informed, but the patient himself was kept in the dark, even though, in most instances, he knew the truth anyway. "It was like there was some magical belief that if you didn't say the word cancer, it was not true. People would whisper the word or call it 'the big C.'"

Goldbloom cites another seemingly small but hugely significant aspect of the art of medicine: the ability to remain silent and listen. Studies show the average length of time it takes a doctor to interrupt a patient is 12 seconds. "Imagine, you go to see your physician for the first time and even before you've begun, he or she has interrupted you."

Compare that, he says, with how communication was handled in years past. Both Goldbloom's father and grandfather were pediatricians. His father, Richard, once wrote an essay called "The Lost Art of Consultation — Let's Dust Off the Old Striped Trousers," which recalled the style of consultation used by his father, Alton. In those days, Alton Goldbloom practised out of an office on Montreal's Crescent Street. If he was seeing a patient for the first time, he would invite the parents, the sick child and their family doctor to meet with him in conference. Then, he and the family doctor would retire to a private salon to discuss the case in more detail, before returning to present their joint findings to the family.

"That," Goldbloom acknowledges, represented "optimal communication." Today, a consultant physician often gets a one-sentence referral letter saying that the patient has pain, please assess and treat. "So you examine the patient and send a report to the referring doctor and never have a face-to-face conversation or even a phone call."

It's unlikely that the profession will ever return to the older model, Goldbloom concedes. Similarly, it's unlikely to arrest the continuing trend toward subspecialization. "A subspecialist," he quips, "is someone who knows more and more about less and less. You can't reverse that steam engine and it's necessary to advance knowledge."

But what it also necessitates, he says, is the supervisory role of the primary care physician, someone able to quarterback and integrate the work of a team that may include half a dozen or more specialists.

When he is ill himself, Goldbloom visits Toronto internist Howard Abrams. "I consider him a great doctor. Why? Because when he examines me, I feel examined in a good way. He makes me feel like he has all the time in world for me, like I am his only patient. He's never preoccupied. He listens. And there is something so relieving in knowing that an experienced physician has laid hands on you. It's extraordinarily comforting."

More than most medical fields, he maintains, psychiatry is cloistered in secrecy, "so people get away with things they might not in other areas. But there's a reason operating theatres are called theatres. It's a theatre. They used to have stadium seating." When his father-in-law taught family psychiatry at the Jewish General Hospital in Montreal, he would do demonstrations for students every week in an auditorium, in front of 200 people, showing how to interview entire families.

On occasion, Epstein would interview healthy families with no dysfunction, just to trip up his students. That, says Goldbloom, is "an important reminder that doctors will see patients who are fundamentally healthy, and that part of the art of medicine and part of being a doctor is to reassure people that they are healthy."

His own father used to describe the practice of pediatrics as the "treatment of anxious parents of healthy children." Frequently, when parents brought a child suffering from headaches, the pediatrician would say, "'In my experience, it's not uncommon in these situations for one or both parents to fear the child might have a brain tumour.' At which point one or the other parent would burst into tears."

The point, says Goldbloom, is that part of any doctor's mission is "to expose the hidden agenda. And that's as true in internal medicine as it is in psychiatry."

What future generations of doctors need more of, Goldbloom suggests, is time observing clinicians at work. "What students clamour for is independence, especially in doing procedures. But they spend less time observing someone taking a history. After all, the physical exam simply confirms what you should know from taking a good history, and that's the art of listening and synthesizing."

When working with his own students, final year residents in psychiatry, Goldbloom makes a practice of doing a complete assessment of patients every four or five weeks, while they observe. Many of them, he says, "may not have seen a full assessment performed in three years. That to me is an indictment of our educational system, but I'm a voice in the wilderness."

CHAPTER 3

LESSONS *of*
the MONTREAL YEARS

He who studies medicine without books sails an uncharted sea,
but he who studies medicine without patients does not go to
sea at all.
— Sir William Osler

THE HARD DECISION TO EMIGRATE having been made, I now faced another thorny question: where exactly to go. A number of friends and colleagues had happily moved to the United States, and I did receive a few informal American overtures. But my first preference was Canada, which I judged to be a gentler society.

Accordingly, I sent letters of introduction to the chiefs of medicine at hospitals in several major Canadian cities. General internists were not in high demand at the time, so I was not exactly deluged with offers. But I did receive replies about potential positions in Halifax, Edmonton and St. John's. I made a visit to Ottawa, but was discouraged by the February snowbanks that literally reached to the eaves of houses. And one Toronto physician-in-chief expressed interest, but with a caveat: he wanted me to effectively audition in private practice for a few years before applying for a staff position.

Then I received a one-line response from Montreal's McGill University, offering — sight unseen — to make me an assistant professor of medicine and consulting physician at the Royal Victoria Hospital. I waited one week and then accepted, without ever having set foot in Montreal. I arrived with my family in September 1973, a period of resurgent French nationalism in Quebec. A new adventure was about to begin.

Our first weeks were spent in the Royal Terrace Hotel, not far from St. Joseph's Oratory, one of Montreal's famous landmarks. One day I took the family for a walk. Along the way, we met a francophone priest and stopped to chat. Noticing that my daughter was wearing a winter coat, even though it was still only September, he said, "You must be visitors."

We explained who we were and why we had come.

"Welcome," he declared with genuine enthusiasm. "As Jamaicans, you and we Québécois are fellow sufferers of colonialism. I'm glad you did not go to Ontario."

The faculty I joined at McGill was among the world's most distinguished. Its extraordinary constellation of medical talent included endocrinologist John Beck, chairman of the department; Arthur Vineberg, the father of coronary artery surgery, famous for the invention of the Vineberg procedure, a precursor of cardiac bypass operations today; nephrologist John Dirks; endocrinologist Max McKenzie; hematologist Bernie Cooper and future palliative care specialist and nephrologist John Seely. John Meakins was to be my service chief and Peter Paré (who co-authored the Fraser and Paré chest radiology textbook, *Diagnosis of Diseases of the Chest*) was my unofficial guardian. I also remember fondly Martin Hoffman, at once a great physician and superb orator.

In earlier years, the renowned Wilder Penfield, Montreal's famed neurosurgeon and founder of the Montreal Neurological Institute and Hospital, had also taught there, as had anesthesiologist John Sanderson (he'd previously been head of anesthesiology and the founder of the intensive care unit at the University Hospital in Jamaica), the legendary Sir William Osler and Norman Bethune. At that time, McGill ranked ahead of even Harvard or Johns Hopkins and produced genuine five-star physicians. More than a dozen future chiefs of medicine emerged from this extraordinary environment, taking their expertise to the wider world. For me, a mere country doctor from Jamaica, it was very heady stuff.

When I arrived in Montreal, I quickly made an appointment to see the chief of medicine, Dr. John Beck — who, like 20 percent of the staff, was an American.

"We're very pleased to have you here, Dr. Ho," he said.

"And I'm very pleased to be here. But tell me — what exactly is my job description?"

"Well," he said, "the truth is, we don't actually have a job description for you."

It was an odd arrangement, but entirely to my liking, allowing me to do what I thought I might do best — serve as a consulting general physician (known as a general internist in North America).

Two weeks later, I found myself supervising ward rounds with a group of residents, interns and medical students. At University Hospital in Jamaica (and most of the British Commonwealth), it had been the custom during rounds to actually spend time with the patient; in Montreal I found the team would simply gather in the corridor with the patient's file and discuss the case.

Outside one room, the resident informed me that this particular patient was a candidate for a liver biopsy.

"Perhaps, I should examine him then," I said, "since that's a potentially dangerous procedure."

"That won't be necessary," the resident assured me. "We examined him this morning."

"Look," I said, "where I come from, we examine patients. Give me 30 seconds."

So I examined him and, a minute later, declared that the liver they were about to biopsy was, in fact, a kidney. A murmur of surprise buzzed through the group.

"What did he say? What did he say?"

"I said, this mass is a kidney, not a liver. It's a very large kidney and we need to find out why."

"How do you know?"

"I know because that is what a kidney feels like. Where is the intravenous pyelogram?" I asked, referring to the gold standard imaging procedure for the kidney during that era.

"Rounds are finished until this afternoon," the chief resident promptly announced. An hour later, he emerged with the imaging result (IVP) confirming that it was indeed a kidney.

The story of this clinical encounter quickly spread through the Royal Victoria Hospital and the rest of the McGill system. This served as a much-needed impetus for significant changes in the teaching of clinical medicine in Montreal and the rest of Canada — the re-introduction of bedside teaching in the curriculum in those institutions that had discontinued this traditional approach.

Just how urgently reform was needed was borne out by a 1978 paper written for the *Journal of Medical Education*. It reported that while many physicians on rounds believed that they were spending considerable time teaching at patient bedsides, videotapes of these encounters indicated that, in fact, they were doing so only 16 percent of the time. For half the time, the presence of the patient was gratuitous. Most rounds were conducted in corridors, where medical students often confessed to being inattentive or having trouble hearing the teaching physician.

In time, I was able to change the way rounds were conducted at the Royal Victoria Hospital. Thereafter, they took place in the presence of patients with bedside examinations, where necessary.

I had been in Montreal a number of years when Gilbert, a 50-year-old star detective from the city's police force, appeared in my office. He was somewhat pale, complained of backache and had experienced a modest weight loss (less than 10 pounds). Physicians he had already seen suggested his problem was essentially mechanical, likely disc-related, and thought he might qualify for workmen's compensation.

Now, it was my turn for a little detective work. Although Gilbert's hemoglobin level was normal, his erythrocyte sedimentation rate (ESR) — the rate at which red blood cells tend to adhere — was 80. Normal would be less than 15. A high ESR rate is commonly taken to indicate the presence of inflammation in the body and can be an early clue to potentially serious organic disease.

That reading led me to the hypothesis that he could have a serious disease. I suspected multiple myeloma, a blood cancer arising from the bone marrow. Further testing, including protein electrophoresis and examination of the bone marrow, confirmed the diagnosis.

In the subsequent weeks and months, I came to know Gilbert quite well. One day, he appeared as a subject/patient case study for a clinic I was leading for a group of six medical students. I pointed out to them, as I always did, the value of observation — taking note, for example, of the importance of examining a patient's neck veins as potential indicia of cardio-vascular illness.

The detective stopped me right there.

"What you are doing is exactly the way I train my rookie detectives," he said. "It's all about paying attention to what you see."

Then, spontaneously, we devised a little experiment. We asked the students to close their eyes and tell us what objects were in the room. Most could accurately name only two or three out of 10. Then we let them keep their eyes open for two minutes and actively observe the objects in the room and repeated the test. Not surprisingly, by focussing harder, we recorded a five-fold increase in the number of items observed.

This was an important lesson, both for me and for them — not just to "see" or look at something passively, but to "look at it" actively. Sadly, although his illness was treatable, it was not curable. Gilbert succumbed to the disease a few years later. But three decades later, I am still using that same experiment with students.

And as I suggested in my Introduction, the same approach applies to hearing and touch.

Instead of just hearing (passive), physicians must listen (active). Instead of just feeling a lump in the neck, they must learn to palpate it. Ask yourself: this lump — how big is it? Is it hard or soft? What lies beside it? Is there a relationship to the surrounding tissue? Does it disappear if we change the head's position? Is it draining into the lymph nodes? These questions will help make the examination a more active process.

Similarly, with a heart murmur: what am I listening for? How loud is the murmur? What is its character? Does it change with respiration? Does it radiate in any direction? A sharper focus on what you are doing will almost certainly improve diagnostic accuracy.

I part company here with journalist Malcolm Gladwell's argument in his book *Outliers: The Story of Success* that great expertise is only acquired after 10,000 hours of experience. A good physician only needs to have seen a condition once before to commit its characteristics to informed memory, and to be able to diagnose it correctly if he or she encounters it again.

You have to develop effectively two separate skill sets — the intuitive talent of Sherlock Holmes, and the harder, more scientific approach of Dr. Watson.

I recall one Montreal case in which both observation and deduction were required. While on teaching rounds, my students and I came across Eleanor, a very sick 30-year-old woman. She had high fever, shortness of breath and tremor. It appeared to me to be a probable case of staphylococcus aureus septicemia (a blood infection). Physicians consider it the "cancer" of microbial agents because it spreads as quickly and as widely (metastasizing) as some aggressive cancers. Untreated, it can be lethal within two or three days.

As I was examining her, I noticed a series of four or five little dots, like puncture wounds, on her leg, just above the ankle.

"Where did you get those?" I asked.

"Oh," Eleanor replied. "I fell off my bicycle and the parts of the chain stabbed me."

I peered more closely at the wounds. The story was certainly plausible, but I suspected something else. The marks on her leg weren't sufficiently uniform, in shape or alignment, to have been caused by the bicycle's chain.

"Where are your needles?"

The young woman immediately started to cry and, soon after, confessed to injecting herself with drugs (via the saphenous or leg vein). The contaminated heroin she was injecting had quickly been carried to the right side of the heart, formed a bacterial non-cancerous growth (a vegetation) on the valve, and subsequently embolized to the lungs, where it produced abscesses. I was thus able to say right then that she was suffering from staphylococcus endocarditis, a bacterial infection of the heart's lining. This is sometimes known as tricuspid endocarditis, common in places with high numbers of intravenous drug users. Fortunately for Eleanor, it was curable with antibiotics.

Inevitably, if you practise long enough, you will meet patients who lie in other ways. I recall the quiet of one Sunday morning in the emergency ward in Montreal disturbed by rising concern about Victor, a young man, also about 30, who worked in the hospital's emergency ward.

The chart showed that he was running a consistent fever of exactly 104.3 degrees and experiencing violent rigours, or whole body chills, as well as an accelerated heart rate and some blood in his urine. The ER doctors had already started him on a course of antibiotics, having diagnosed pyelonephritis, an infection of the urinary tract. Untreated, the condition could lead to septicemia and death.

I approached the bed, where Victor lay shaking violently under the white bed sheet (actually too violently, as you will see).

"Are you ready for this?" I asked the doctors and nurses gathered around me. And with that, I suddenly yanked the bed sheet away from him and flung it on the floor. Simultaneously we heard the sound of glass hitting the concrete floor — *clinkety, clink, clink, clink* — a set of eight thermometers, all registering at exactly 104.3 degrees!

Deeply embarrassed, Victor promptly got up, dressed and left the hospital.

Although I had taken a risk with my dramatic approach to exposing him, I'd never seen a case where, in six consecutive readings, the temperature was always the same. That was the clue that this illness was not what it seemed. If you take a patient's temperature over a period of several hours, almost invariably, there will be slight variations. His were static, a straight line. Moreover, shaking chills or rigours are usually not as violent as this patient's shaking: his were like the violent shaking in a grand mal seizure attack.

This was a clear case of factitious fever, which is sometimes related to Munchausen syndrome. Its name derives from 18th-century German nobleman Baron Münchhausen, who had a great gift for embellishing the truth. The medical syndrome was named formally by British endocrinologist Richard Asher in 1951, to describe situations in which people fabricate histories, signs and symptoms of illness to get admitted to hospital.

In Victor's case, he had faked his body chills, fixed the temperature settings on the thermometers (by immersing all eight thermometers in hot water at the same time) and pricked his finger with a stylet to create blood in the urine. We later found the stylet that he used to prick his finger in the night table drawer beside his bed.

NOT ALL APPARENT MYSTERIES, OF course, are so easily solved. One day, I was visited by Merle, a woman of about 34, who'd been referred by a family physician. She had a history of eye problems and was now complaining of fatigue and a general sense of unease. Her hemoglobin was 150 (normal is 120–130) — a possible indication of polycythemia, a disproportionate rise in the blood's red cells.

Six weeks later, Merle returned, still feeling unwell, with a hemoglobin reading of 160. More time passed, and the reading continued to climb, to 180. By then there were subtle differences in her neurological exam — i.e., minor changes in the tremor of her fingers on testing for coordination. This indicated a problem in her cerebellum, which is the part of the brain essential for normal coordination and balance. That minor signal — and the hemoglobin readings — got my attention. A high hemoglobin count is commonly caused by low oxygen levels. These can be caused either by chronic lung disease or shunts in the heart that divert blood from the lungs.

A high hemoglobin count can also be caused by excess erythropoietin, which is essential for the production of hemoglobin. It is erythropoietin (epo) that has often been used — and abused — by professional athletes, especially cyclists, long-distance runners, speed skaters and cross-country skiers for blood doping, to increase oxygen-rich red cell counts. Many sports organizations have officially banned it, most famously the Tour de France and the Olympics.

Though rare, certain tumours can also produce erythropoietin in excess and thus cause high hemoglobin. There were only a few possibilities, among them renal cell carcinoma, or kidney cancer; thymoma; fibroids; liver cancer or a rare brain tumour, a cerebellar hemangioblastoma. A subsequent brain scan revealed the tumour, situated in her cerebellum (cerebellar hemangioblastoma).

Fortunately, the tumour could be removed by surgery and the young woman was able to fully recover. How rare is a cerebellar hemangioblastoma? I have not seen it since, which may help explain why the details of the case remain so vivid in my memory.

What I did see again, three decades later, was another case that involved elevated red blood cell counts. This time, the patient was a 68-year-old Asian woman who complained of mild headaches, fatigue, high blood pressure and a history of asthma. Her mucous membrane had a slightly reddish hue, which was explained by her hemoglobin reading — 180. The asthma suggested an oxygen deficiency, which can drive up hemoglobin levels. We commonly see this in patients with serious lung disease; in such cases, hemoglobin counts may be as high as 200, but her examination and tests for asthma were all normal.

Recalling the Montreal case from years before, I ordered a CT scan of the cerebellum, but there was no evidence of tumour. Other scans showed no lung damage, no abdominal tumours and no cirrhosis of the liver. Her erythropoietin level in the blood was high. The question that perplexed me was what explained the elevated levels of epo?

Then I remembered that an ultrasound of the abdomen does not include the pelvis. A CT scan was ordered and a benign, grapefruit-sized fibroid was discovered. That was the source of her erythropoietin. It had made her blood too thick — the cause of her headaches and general fatigue and difficulty concentrating. A hysterectomy, removing the fibroid, cured her.

DURING MY EARLY YEARS IN Montreal in the 1970s, we did not yet have access to sophisticated ultrasound or CT technology. This made diagnoses more complicated, and I occasionally resorted to distinctly unconventional approaches. McGill, at that time, maintained a close medical relationship with the University of Nairobi. Personnel went back and forth regularly, working on aspects of infectious disease.

On one occasion, a colleague of mine returned from Kenya with a persistent fever. He was sweating frequently and losing weight, but tests ruled out both malaria and typhoid fever. My instinct was that he had developed a liver abscess, caused by amoebae he may have consumed in the Kenyan drinking water. To test my theory, I actually punched him — lightly — in the liver. His pained reaction told me I was right. We quickly drained the abscess, administered antibiotics and he made a complete recovery. Today, ultrasound or CT scans make diagnosis of these lesions precise, but you still have to make the clinical diagnosis before ordering those tests.

Some three decades later, I received a call from a family physician, Dr. David Greenberg, who asked me to examine one of his patients, a desperately ill man of about 50. He came in with fever and chills, slightly jaundiced. I punched him — not too hard — in the liver and, based on his wincing reaction, was convinced he had a liver abscess. I sent him for an ultrasound the same day, which confirmed the diagnosis.

Despite the time it requires, the critical importance of documenting a patient's full history — personal and professional — was underscored to me in one fascinating Montreal case. Two members of the city's police department paid me a visit. They did not come to interrogate me. They came separately, each describing a similar set of symptoms — decreased appetites, mild abdominal pain and reduced energy levels. The malaise was non-specific; they just didn't feel quite right. When I saw them, each had been ill for more than six months. Curiously, I learned, they had often worked together.

Even though I had no indication of why, one of the early differential diagnoses was lead poisoning. After a series of non-conclusive tests on the first patient, we decided to test lead levels in his blood. They proved to be far above the normal range. So the diagnosis was now clear: lead poisoning. The question was why.

Lead plays an interesting role in the history of disease. Affecting several organs and tissues, toxic levels can produce symptoms that range from mild confusion and abdominal pain to coma and death. Its effects were observed as early as the second century BC by the Greek botanist Nicander, who described its consumption as leading to colic and paralysis. Some academics maintain that lead, used widely in Roman aqueducts for 800 years, may have contributed to the fall of the Roman Empire, its toxins seeping into the water supply via lead plumbing.

In the modern era, lead mixed into paint has been blamed for lead poisoning in children. Children and adults exposed to lead poisoning typically show impaired intellectual ability.

In the 1980s, Canadian researchers conducted tests on the cadavers of victims of the ill-fated Franklin expeditions of the 19th century, British explorers famously lost in the Arctic. Examination of their bones revealed lead content of 228 parts per million, versus only 22–36 ppm in the bones of Native Canadians accompanying the mission. The villain: cans of meat (bully beef) that the explorers had stocked on board their ships. The tins were the product of a then novel technology, soldered by lead and tin.

I doubted whether that was the cause of lead levels in the blood of the first police officer who came to me, but something was.

As I often do, I began with a few questions about his work.

"You're a policeman, I see."

"Yes."

"How long have you been on the force?"

"Twenty years."

"Do you live near a battery-making plant or a battery dump?"

Lead in such waste facilities has been known to leech into the water supply.

"No," he said.

"What are your responsibilities on the force?"

"I've done various things, but for several years I taught other officers how to shoot guns."

"At an outdoor shooting range?"

"Indoors. And underground."

Bingo, as they say. The air in that subterranean facility would have been filled with microscopic fragments of lead. My patient would have breathed it into his lungs every day and had it on his hands when he ate lunch. Repeated exposure had produced the effects of lead poisoning.

When his colleague came to see me with similar symptoms, that mystery was even more quickly resolved. He had also spent many hours in the indoor shooting range.

Both men were successfully treated with the drug, dimercaprol, which leeches lead out of the system via the urine.

So while it is sometimes suggested that getting to know your patient is a waste of time, my own experience is that it is essential. At a minimum, it helps cement the connection between doctor and patient, establishing a bond of trust likely to make treatment more effective. And, as with the Montreal police officers, it can yield the answer to the origins of disease and distress.

ONE DAY IN MONTREAL, I was asked to attend to Colette, a 79-year-old woman who had broken her arm. Apparently, she had been kneeling in church, at prayer, when she collapsed, falling onto her limb. We started chatting and she related the terrible experience. I took her pulse — a normal 70 beats per minute. Then I put my finger on her carotid sinus, located in the neck just below the angle of the jaw. The pace was 40 beats per minute, a disturbingly low pace. Carotid sinus pressure can cause the heart to slow, by increasing what is known as the vagal tone (relating to the vagus nerve).

By chance, visiting my office was Dr. Maurice McGregor, a professor of cardiology and at that time the chief of medicine at Royal Victoria Hospital.

"What are you doing?" he asked.

I explained that I had just examined an elderly patient who had fallen in church, broken her arm, had a very slow pulse and was likely suffering from what is known as carotid sinus syndrome, the cause of her syncope or fainting spell. She probably needed to have a pacemaker implanted in her heart, I suggested.

"I don't believe you," he said. "Let me have a look."

Together, we went to visit the patient. McGregor placed his fingers on her carotid artery. Now, the heart rate was 38 beats per minute.

Still, he was unconvinced. "This doesn't prove anything, Herbert."

"Maybe not, but do you want to wait until it's 30 and she falls and breaks a hip?" I think he was annoyed that I was telling him, a cardiologist, what needed to be done.

Finally, with a twinkle in his eye, he graciously conceded the point. McGregor was no ordinary cardiologist. He later went on to integrate South Africa's Witwatersrand medical school, even before the release of Nelson Mandela.

Sometimes known as Stokes-Adams attacks, cardiac syncope is not rare. The cause may be electrical — the heart's natural pacemaker may fail, leading to heart block (i.e., a very slow heart rate). Or it may beat too fast. It can also be mechanical, precipitated by organic disease of some kind, aortic valve stenosis or hypertropic cardiomyopathy. If the heart beats too slowly (30 beats per minute or less), not enough blood flows to the brain, so it shuts down the system and you faint. If the heart beats too fast — say, 200 beats per minute — the same thing will happen. On occasion, the beat may alternate between too fast and too slow in the same person, the so-called tachybrady syndrome.

In a typical cardiac syncope episode, everything is fine until it isn't. You lose balance then consciousness, usually leading to a fall to the floor and, frequently, injuries. This is part of what distinguishes it from vasovagal attacks, which usually come with some warning — dizziness, nausea or tinnitus (ringing in the ears). Epilepsy may also induce syncope, though again there are distinguishing features such as flashing lights (prodrome) or twitching. Or you may have a grand mal seizure, usually followed by disorientation.

Physicians must therefore be careful to determine which form of syncope they are treating. With cardiac syncope, recovery — if you survive — is usually spontaneous, with full memory of the event. Regardless, it is critically important to understand the precise circumstances that led to syncope because it is a potentially serious and life-threatening problem.

Jeremy, a man of about 45, came to see me after fainting on a beautiful summer day at his cottage. He was sitting on a dock by the lake when, without warning, he suddenly fainted. It lasted only 25 seconds and then he came to. He thought he had fallen asleep.

I saw Jeremy a few months later and he seemed otherwise healthy. We did an echocardiogram and outfitted him with a Holter, a monitor that measures and records the heart's electrical competence. The latter told us he was suffering from intermittent but complete heart block in the conduction system. In lay terms, his wiring was defective. Causes of this potentially lethal condition include coronary artery disease, fibrosis or sarcoidosis, a non-infectious TB-like illness. Jeremy needed a pacemaker, which corrected the problem.

So did Fern, a 42-year-old woman who fainted while driving, crashing her car into a tree. Shaken but not badly injured, she went to an emergency room. Tests there turned up nothing definitive, and she was then sent to a neurologist to see if the blackout had been caused by epileptic seizure. Again, her brain function was normal. At that point, they asked for my opinion. I took her history, which included a bout of sarcoidosis some 15 years earlier. We outfitted her with a Holter, which proved normal, but an MRI revealed a lesion on her left ventricle.

Her history of pulmonary sarcoid, the syncopal event and the MRI of her heart showing the nodule all suggested susceptibility to heart block and the need for a pacemaker. One was implanted and Fern has experienced no recurrence of syncope.

The pacemaker, in most cases, can successfully address problems of syncope caused by brachycardia (heart beating too slowly). But it should be remembered that the pacemaker, too, is a machine and can malfunction, adding complications. And not every incident of cardiac syncope needs to be treated with a pacemaker.

Lawrence, an Anglican priest of about 64 years, had experienced recurrent syncopal episodes for a year. His palpitations and flushing were so severe that he had rushed off to an emergency room on four or five occasions. Cardiologists and internal medicine specialists had examined and tested him with electrocardiograms, an echocardiogram and a Holter device, but were unable to find any organic problem.

When I saw him, he complained that his tachycardia was making his life miserable.

"Tell me," I said, "are you high church Anglican or low church?"

"High church," he said.

In the high church, priests take communion, the symbolic re-enactment of the Last Supper, by eating a wafer and drinking wine.

I said, "Maybe you are having these attacks because you are allergic to the sulfites in red wine. Stop drinking it completely and see what happens."

For the first year, Lawrence had no further attacks. But after that, every now and then, he would attend a celebration and drink a glass of wine, beer or half a glass of champagne — and another attack would ensue. But as long as he remained abstinent, he was fine.

BOTH PERSONALLY AND PROFESSIONALLY, my 10 years in Montreal were happy and successful. But by the early 1980s, I was in my early 40s: if I were ever going to make another career move, it was certainly the time.

Dr. BRIAN HODGES

Brian Hodges graduated from Queen's University School of
Medicine in 1989, completed a psychiatry residency at the
University of Toronto in 1994, a master's of Higher Education in
1995 and a Ph.D. in 2007. Since 2003, he has been the director of
the University of Toronto Wilson Centre, one of the largest centres
for health professional education research in the world. From
2004 to 2008, he was chair of evaluation at the Royal College of
Physicians and Surgeons of Canada, overseeing assessment of the 62
specialty programs. He was named full professor and the Richard
and Elizabeth Currie chair in Health Professions Education
Research at University of Toronto in 2009 and vice president
education at the University Health Network (UHN) in 2010.

IT'S LIKELY THAT FEW PHYSICIANS are more in sync with the
teaching philosophy of Dr. Herbert Ho Ping Kong than Dr. Brian
Hodges, the University Health Network's vice president for education. In various roles, he has spent the last 20 years trying to incul-
cate the principles of humane practice. Just how essential they
have become in an age of transcendent technologies was brought
home to him a few years ago: he became a patient in his own hospital system when he suffered a ruptured appendix while on the job.

"I would say my own experience was mixed," he says, reflect-
ing on the event. "I didn't know it was happening to me. There
were some good clinical skills on display, but there was also a little bit of 'let's see what the CT scanner says' kind of thinking. And
appendicitis is still a clinical diagnosis, by and large."

The incident, Hodges says, solidified his conviction that educators must be careful not to "deskill in the art and humane practice side of medicine."

More than psychiatry, he says, medicine needs "to continue to emphasize the physical examination and basic clinical skills. What I love about Herbert's message is that he makes the case that medicine rests on the basic contact between patient and doctor. But there's no doubt we have drifted away from it." Hodges' own specialty, psychiatry, is not exempt from these principles.

Although most of Hodges' time is now devoted to administration, when he's on call, he heads for the emergency ward. His first question to residents is "'Which patients have had a physical exam?' And if they haven't done it, I'll say, 'Let's go do it.' Sometimes they'll look at me like I have three heads. But until you've done a comprehensive clinical assessment, you don't know anything about anybody."

Advocates for the traditional patient-centric approach, Hodges concedes, often confront a challenge from other doctors — the argument that there is not sufficient evidence to justify huge expenditures of time interviewing patients when technology, in the form of the CT scan or an ultrasound machine, can often do a better diagnostic job.

It was in part to answer such critiques, he says, that "Herbert set up his Centre for Education in Excellence and Practice [CEEP] at Toronto Western, to conduct research that would not only prove the value of the physical exam, but demonstrate that the empathic relationship formed between doctor and patient pays health dividends. There's some great work in diabetes that shows that people with strong doctor-patient bonds live longer and have better outcomes. So he's using science, evidence-based medicine, to prove his case."

The MRI, CT scanner and other marvels of technology represent a great set of tools, he allows. "But if you are building a house, you don't start with the circular saw. You start with a plan, with a design. We could send every person in the emergency room to get a CT scan when they arrived, but there is no brain activity for that. It's like trying to build a house without an architect, without a plan."

And no single machine — or even constellation of machines — he notes, can do pattern recognition the way a human can. "And pattern recognition remains the heart of diagnostic medicine. It rests entirely on a doctor sitting down with a patient, looking at them, listening to them, talking to them, assembling the story and then using the technological tools as an adjunct to confirm suspicions or a hypothesis."

In Hodges' experience, medical students in their early years broadly accept the importance of learning and practising the art of medicine. Often, it's a validation of the idealistic thinking that may have brought them to the profession in the first place. But as they move through the system, they become exposed to the so-called hidden curriculum, which begins to undo their instincts and hardens them.

"Remember that as third- and fourth-year students, as clinical clerks, they not only see humane, caring role models like Herbert and his disciples," says Hodges. "They see other faculty members who take shortcuts and look for efficiencies. And they see conflicts between different medical services over what constitutes the right approach or what's important. If it's not handled well, the student begins to stop doing things they once did, because he's hearing that it's not really important. And if too many of those factors impinge at the same time, they may take a very rudimentary approach and fall into the trap of relying on technology, or stop thinking — just refer the problem to someone else."

In fact, he says, it's a fallacy that humane medicine takes a huge amount of time. "Being empathic and making a connection does not take an hour. My best role model for this, when I was an intern, was actually a surgeon. I was at Toronto's St. Joseph's Hospital and in those days, we had short three-week rotations. He sat down with me and said, 'Brian, most of my patients are dying of cancer and we only have about five minutes with each of them, but you must make a connection with them in that time. Yes, the x-rays are important. Yes, the follow-up is important.

The time is short, but there's no reason you can't build a relationship in five minutes.' And he was absolutely right."

Is there a protocol to follow in the process? Absolutely, says Hodges. "Rule number one would be not to look at your watch."

Not long ago, an advocate from Toronto General Hospital's office of patient relations related an instructive anecdote to Hodges. A doctor walked into a patient's room and immediately began talking. The patient interrupted him and said, "Excuse me, would you mind if we began by you telling me who you are, and I'll tell you who I am, and we can chat for a minute before discussing what my MRI says?" The doctor apologized and said, "Of course, you are right." "So a lot of this is simple human communication skills," says Hodges.

Nothing is going to change the current paradigm of subspecialization, Hodges believes, but "if I'm a diabetes specialist or if I only treat patients with schizophrenia, or if I deal with post-partum hemorrhage, I need to constantly remind myself that medicine is larger than this. A lot of the responsibility rests on those who train subspecialists — to challenge them to understand the generalist's perspective and communicate their thoughts to the generalist, which is often the family practitioner." But there are, he acknowledges, weaknesses in the system. "There need to be more conversations. The specialists have to reach out to the generalists and say, 'What do you think? You know the whole person.'"

To counteract the tendency to reductionism, the subspecialist has to approach the patient and his or her family with humility, Hodges contends. "The opening conversation should not be about the blood sugar levels but 'How are you? What's the big picture?'"

Every patient, he says, is a unique canvas and thus requires a custom-made approach. "The art in the art of medicine is not just a generic 'be nice to people.' It's like any other art, a set of refined skills that can be learned and need mentorship and modelling. How I talk to someone in the emergency ward who is depressed is quite different than how I'd talk to someone who is dying and needs palliative care."

The medical historian Edward Shorter, Hodges says, has documented the decline of the art of medicine. "There was more art when there was less science and fewer drugs, when doctors made house calls and saw patients in their homes. We've slid from that longitudinal relationship." Now, some medical schools are attempting to revive the longitudinal approach, with students spending a year with one mentor/doctor, instead of two weeks.

Hodges himself chairs the management committee of the Phoenix Project, a multi-year initiative that aims to give doctors and nurses a better balance between human compassion and technical expertise. The project was launched by the charity Associated Medical Services, which felt medicine was drifting away from the model of compassionate care. If that care were measured today on a scale of 10, our current performance, Hodges maintains, would be below average.

"A lot of it is our fault," he says. "Medical students come in with those values and we undo them in our institutions. You can make people better or worse, depending on the environment they work in."

AN

INFECTIOUS DISEASE SPECIALIST'S

PERSPECTIVE

Dr. DAVID McNEELY

Dr. David McNeely is an internist, consultant in infectious diseases at the University Health Network and an associate professor of medicine at the University of Toronto.

THERE CANNOT BE MANY DOCTORS who can claim what David McNeely can claim — that in the same hospital, Toronto Western, he was born, became a medical student, then an intern, then a chief resident and, after a two-year fellowship in infectious diseases at the University of Florida (Gainesville), a practitioner for more than 35 years.

The son of a customs and excise officer, McNeely said his father — frustrated by working within a large, top-down bureaucracy — urged his three sons to choose a profession that would help them avoid such structural impotence. His two brothers chose law. McNeely chose medicine.

As he neared completion of his chief residency, McNeely still wasn't certain which subspeciality he wanted to pursue. Toronto Western's then physician-in-chief Abraham Rapoport helped him decide.

"He told me, 'I don't need another cardiologist. I do need someone in infectious disease.' Cardiology is mechanical. Your whole life becomes three vessels and one disease, essentially. Rapoport wanted someone with catholic knowledge and that suited me. I never regretted it. I got to interact with all kinds of disciplines and wasn't just a left lobe of the thyroid guy."

When McNeely departed for Gainesville in the late 1970s, there was only one infectious disease specialist in Toronto. Today, there are 60. The numbers testify to the recognition that the world we inhabit is essentially made up of man and microbes.

Mostly, says McNeely, we live symbiotically. "We adapt or develop immunity. But some creatures are not as friendly and have the potential to invade us." And everywhere but the First World, death by microbe is "still the most common way to exit the planet. Two children in five in the Third World die before their fifth birthday, usually from infectious diarrhea or malaria."

Given what he calls the growing "armamentarium of technology," McNeely argues that the art of medicine is "increasingly relevant." In theory, he maintains, we could now give a series of algorithms to a bright high-school student — sequencing patient complaints, lab test analyses and the latest evidence guidelines — and "as long as they followed the logic, line by line — the serum ginger ale, the stool rhubarb, the total body MRI — they could take a pretty good cut at diagnosis. That's the science. But is that satisfactory for the patient or for society or even intellectually for the practitioner?"

What is missing is the art of medicine, "taking the human condition in all its variations into consideration. What is the average rate of compliance with pharmaceutics in non-symptomatic conditions? How many people with high blood pressure are actually taking their medication? The answer is it is highly variable and depends on a host of things, not least your relationship with your doctor. But the bottom line is if you get 75 percent, you are doing well. And in some communities, it's 50 percent. Is that the best you can do? Well, if you want to do better, the solution is not in the computer. It's in the art of medicine. It's needed at all levels, but the earlier in the process you are, and the broader your involvement with the patient, the greater the necessity. If your doctor is a catheterizing cardiologist or an anesthetist or a colorectal surgeon, you hope he or she is humane, but the art component is less critical, as long as they are iron-clad competent."

McNeely credits Dr. Herbert Ho Ping Kong with restoring the key role played by the general internist — an academic generalist with comprehensive knowledge of many disciplines. That need, he says, has grown as the aging population presents more and more cases of chronic and simultaneous multi-system disease.

"Remember, the general wards were a professional backwater when he came here from McGill," he says. "The old standard was that if you had heart disease, you saw a cardiologist. If you had renal disease, you saw a nephrologist. If you had diabetes, you saw an endocrinologist. But what if you had all three? Then you dragged yourself around to all of those offices. And if you showed up in the emergency room, there were big battles, not to look after the patient but to send you to the other guy's speciality. And that often led to willful neglect. Herbert was a major instrument of change and de-compartmentalization. Patients, he argued, needed more holistic treatment. You could not arbitrarily decide that Patient X was a heart patient and Patient Y needed a respirologist. And general internists, he said, were well placed to play the role of quarterback. Training had to become more holistic as well. Now it's the paradigm, but then it was a very tough sell, because it meant resources — for beds, for trainees, for dollars, et cetera."

In the more than 30 years since McNeely began practising, he has witnessed dramatic changes in his field — epidemics of Legionnaires' disease, Clostridium difficile, HIV/AIDS and, more recently, SARS. All of it, he suggests, underscores the need to understand our patients, not just their symptoms. "It's not being intrusive," he says. "So many things are defined by whether you have used recreational drugs or a needle, or by your sexual preferences, by your travel, by your behaviour. And, as we hugely advance in technology and hugely advance in informatics, we can't afford to lose sight of the patient. You can't take all your cues from what's on a computer screen. Talk to the patient. We're getting better at it, because the patient is increasingly demanding it. And that's a good thing."

McNeely regards his longtime colleague, Herbert Ho Ping Kong, as a representative of a vanishing breed. "He's a product of a highly traditional and structured British medical school system that does not exist anymore," he says. "And he grew up in the Jesuit school. There were only three instructions — diligence, diligence and diligence. He has the rigour and single-mindedness that only Jesuits have. He is endlessly patient, with every patient he sees. He is empathetic and sympathetic, especially when there is nothing to be done except ameliorate the disease or control its symptoms, as best we can. Finally, he understands that we can have all the technology we want, but we must always keep striving for excellence and we must keep practising, even if we never get perfect."

CHAPTER 4

The ART
of SEEING

*Medicine is learned by the bedside and not in the classroom.
Let not your conceptions of disease come from words heard in
the lecture room or read from the book. See, and then reason
and compare and control. But see first.*

— Sir William Osler

WHEN WE FIRST ARRIVED IN Montreal, my wife and I initially planned to stay for three years, and then assess our professional situation. As it happened, our third anniversary in 1976 roughly coincided with the surprise election of the separatist Parti Québécois, led by the mercurial journalist-turned-politician René Lévesque.

The election results sent the anglophone community in Quebec into a state of shock. I vividly recall walking into Royal Victoria Hospital, at the north end of the McGill University campus, at 9 a.m. on the morning after the election and finding it virtually deserted. The corridors, coffee shops — completely empty. It was as if an official order had been issued to vacate the entire premises.

Virtually no one, it is safe to say, had anticipated the PQ victory, and the ensuing days and weeks were full of discussion about what its election might mean for government policy on a broad range of issues, including health care. Even in those early days, colleagues began to talk out loud about the very real possibility of leaving the province. Tens of thousands of anglophones ultimately ended up doing so, perceiving that in Lévesque's Quebec they would become second-class citizens.

Curiously, perhaps, my wife and I did not seriously consider making an exit. We had both been so happy, personally and professionally, that leaving was not a consideration. Our children were enrolled in excellent schools and had adapted nicely to Canadian culture. Barbara had completed her residency in dermatology and gone into private practice in leafy Westmount, a short walk from our home. She also had a part-time consulting appointment at the Royal Victoria Hospital.

I was busy teaching as an associate professor at McGill University and working as a consulting physician, also at the Royal Victoria Hospital. The administration had allowed me to practise medicine the way I wanted to practise it and to develop my leadership skills. An important mentor for me was Dale Dauphinee, a gastroenterologist who chaired the department's Medical Education Committee and later served as executive director of the Medical Council of Canada.

Dauphinee had a distinct style of management. He was very calm, at once articulate and deliberate. In meetings, his tendency was to sit back and let others lead the discussion. But when a critical issue was on the agenda, or when he felt a poor decision was about to be made, he would sit up and sharply slap his hand on the table and say, "I'm sorry, that's not good enough. We have to do better." It wasn't done in anger, but with firm resolve. That impressed me. He was usually so restrained that on those rare occasions when he decided to exert his authority, it became all the more effective. I tried to model my own managerial performance on those lines, walking softly and carrying a stick that I wielded only when necessary.

All too quickly, it seemed, our three years became five years and then 10. In my capacity as head of the Royal Victoria

1

Hospital's general internal medicine, I was allowed to hire six consecutive chief residents, all of whom went on to enjoy distinguished medical careers. These included Ken Flegel, a consulting internist at the Royal Vic, senior associate editor of the *Canadian Medical Association Journal* and a professor of medicine at McGill; Linda Snell, also a professor of medicine at McGill and senior clinician educator at the Royal College of Physicians and Surgeons of Canada; David Dawson, associate professor of medicine at McGill, an attending physician at the McGill University Health Centre, chief of service of a clinical teaching unit and winner of numerous teaching awards; and Sam Benaroya, recently the acting dean at McGill Medical School.

All of them were from different parts of the country, but they all had graduated, in effect, from the flower child school of philosophy that had been so prevalent during the late 1960s and 1970s. They espoused that more humane approach to practice, even though medicine was then beginning to feel the dramatic impact of several extraordinary technological breakthroughs. In some sense, perhaps, their approach was a reaction to those developments, because these physicians clearly expressed the desire to be more than mere operators of machines, however sophisticated — more than the servants of technology.

"I want," they told me, "to be a doctor that can act on the same patient-driven impulses that made me want to choose medicine as a profession."

I had already established a division of general internal medicine. Within that, I also developed an internal medicine unit (IMU), a model group arrangement in which young physicians were invited to practise collectively, just as they would in private practice. As closely as possible, we tried to mimic the way "private clinics" worked outside the hospital. All of these residents-in-chief and many of their subordinates eventually became part of this unit.

But there were two issues that would ultimately lead Barbara and me to make career changes. The first of these was the political climate that developed in the years that followed the ascension of the so-called Péquistes. We largely learned to live with challenging reforms and budget cutbacks, which became routine. But we were increasingly conscious of the population exodus, particularly of young people, who perceived brighter potentials in Toronto, Western Canada or the United States. It was not a vote of confidence in the future of Quebec.

The other factor was language. To practise in Quebec, we had both needed to demonstrate fluency in French one year after our arrival. My wife had no difficulty with this stipulation, but I did. I had never studied the language and had only the very limited vocabulary necessary for day-to-day interaction with francophones. Thus, not long after settling in at McGill, I enrolled in an instructional class. Given my handicap, I was categorized as a pre-beginner, one of 10 in the class.

The first session was a revelation, conducted entirely in French — immersion. I was completely lost. Five weeks later, halfway through the course, I still had no clear idea what anyone was saying. However, I did manage to understand the teacher when she told me that I was among the most difficult students she had ever had.

"You must be Chinese," she said.

"I'm Jamaican," I protested.

"What language did your parents speak?"

"Chinese."

"Well, that's it, then. That's why you have so much trouble with French."

I was not alone, apparently. A colleague of mine, enrolled in the same class, was taking the pre-beginner's course for the fourth time.

One wintry weekend, Barbara brought home a long-playing record designed to teach French, along with a 50-page booklet. I spent the entire weekend playing the record, studying the book and memorizing vocabulary. By Monday, to my own and others' amazement, I could actually conduct a simple conversation in French.

At our next class, my teacher greeted me with the usual, "*Bon soir, Hebert.*" I responded with a 15-minute monologue in French. I was very proud of myself and my progress — until I took the French exam of the Office Québécois de la langue française (French language test for professionals). The pass mark was 75. I earned a 65. I had failed.

"What am I going to do now?" I asked my wife.

Then I had an idea. I called up the government office that administered the exams. I introduced myself in French and explained everything that had happened. I spoke for 10 minutes. We had a very cordial conversation. The official in charge said to me, "Your French is very good. Why don't you come down to the office for a chat? Come tomorrow. We'll examine you in person." Perhaps he wanted to make sure that I was, in fact, who I said I was.

The next day, I went to see him and an exam board of four others. We spoke in French for 20 minutes, after which he told me in French, "You passed."

Of course, he said it so fast in the heavily accented Québécois style — and my French comprehension was still so rudimentary — that I didn't understand what he had said. He repeated it a few times in French and then finally, when I still was struggling, shouted at me in English, "You passed! You passed!"

In terms of language, then, there was no need for Barbara and me to leave Montreal. We were happily ensconced in a lovely Westmount home, once owned by the president of the Sun Life Insurance Company. And yet, a feeling of linguistic inadequacy continued to nag at me. In internal medicine, you needed to understand and be able to communicate nuances. It's exactly such nuances that constitute a critical part of the art of medicine. And the nuances of Québécois French, I felt, were — and would always be — beyond my ability to master.

The same was true professionally. McGill and the Royal Victoria had given me a wide berth, allowing me to create the internal medicine unit — the first new one in Canada for almost 50 years — and to hire staff.

But I also knew that if I were ever going to leave Montreal, now was probably the right moment. I was in my early 40s, old enough to be considered a seasoned physician, but still young enough to build the next stage of a career. I had become something of an evangelist for the importance of general internal medicine as a distinct discipline, writing for the *Canadian Medical Association Journal* and speaking at 14 medical schools across the country on the topic. And increasingly, the Canadian medical establishment's governing bodies had been willing to embrace that idea.

As a result of these efforts, the Royal College of Physicians and Surgeons subsequently decided to elevate the role of general internal medicine and invited me, under its auspices, to chair a new special committee on internal medicine, with the power to set national standards. I would remain in that position for five years.

In turn, several colleagues and I constructed a Royal College training program geared more directly to general internal medicine, so that it would no longer be an orphaned specialty of the curriculum. Residents in their fourth year could now choose to focus on general internal medicine alone. And we insisted that all residents spend a full year in a clinical teaching unit — a model that had been established by the legendary Sir William Osler. At our discretion, medical schools that did not comply could be awarded only provisional accreditation, the equivalent of a reputational black eye. That gave us some real leverage.

In time, on the recommendation of Edmonton's Dr. Allan Gilbert and its own administrator Ted Gyles, the Royal College also created the Canadian Society of Internal Medicine, with Toronto Western Hospital's Dr. Peter Clark as its first president.

In the meantime, Barbara and I had finally resolved to make a move. I received a very kind offer from the medical school at

McMaster University, but they wanted me to refashion myself as an epidemiologist, which I felt loath to do. I had an equally generous offer from John Dirks, a former colleague of mine at the Royal Vic, who had moved to Vancouver as physician-in-chief and chairman of the department of medicine. It included a staff position and an associate professorship. But during a long courtship, it became clear that Vancouver was not particularly looking for a general internist, and apparently even regarded Dirks, a nephrologist, as something of an outsider. Nor did I feel that Vancouver then was at, or even near, the cutting edge in medicine.

We had already listed our home for sale — my fallback position, if no acceptable offer materialized, was to go into private practice — when Peter Clark called me one morning from Toronto. By the afternoon, we were having coffee in Montreal and he was insisting that I come to Toronto and assume his position as divisional head of general internal medicine. He planned to step down and take a leadership job with Credit Valley, a new hospital under construction west of Toronto. He conceded that he did not yet have formal authorization to make the offer, but assured me that it was just a formality.

He was good to his word. That spring, I accepted Toronto Western's offer to become director of general internal medicine and director of the residency training program. While Clark waited for Credit Valley Hospital to open, he would remain for a year to assist me.

Soon after I accepted the offer to work in Toronto, Montreal's Royal Victoria decided to create a Teacher of the Year Award for the department of medicine. In 1983, this represented a breakthrough for teaching at McGill, where promotion was always based on research and publications (the classic publish or perish philosophy). I was honoured to be designated as the first recipient. But, two days after I was notified of the citation, department officials learned that I had agreed to move to Toronto. They promptly revoked the award. At a subsequent meeting, the dean insisted that he did not want me to leave. But by then it was too late. It was clear to me that despite the creation of the award, teaching — and innovations in teaching — was not considered part of the promotion system at McGill. They were unlikely to bend on this point.

As advocate for general internal medicine, my argument was quite simple. The practice of medicine for the past quarter century had been marked by two dominant features — an explosion of science and technology that began in the late 1950s, and the emergence of medical subspecialties (cardiology, gastroenterology, nephrology, respirology, endocrinology, infectious diseases, etc.).

Indeed, the two went hand in hand because technological innovation made possible new diagnostic tests and equipment that not only extended our tool kits, but required specialists capable of using them and understanding the results. Thus, nephrologists could become experts in dialysis. Cardiologists could master the intricacies of echograms and cardiac catheterizations. Gastroenterologists learned how to use the endoscope for a variety of scoping procedures.

Technology was not only cutting-edge and glamorous; it was rewarding. Government payment schedules effectively encouraged the compartmentalization trend. If physicians performed these procedures, they were paid additional fees. In this environment, specialists in general internal medicine became somewhat marginalized. We were often asked, "What's your role here? What's your specialty?" Not having one became a liability. In a graduating medical class of, say, 60 interns, 58 would typically choose to immerse themselves in a medical subspecialty for their residencies. Part of this was pure pragmatism, because there were far fewer jobs for general internists than for specialists.

These developments, however, were not without consequence, particularly with respect to aging populations and multi-system diseases. If you had chronic lung disease, you saw a respirologist. If you also had a heart condition, you'd also see a cardiologist. If you also had diabetes, then you'd have to see another specialist, an endocrinologist. And if you suffered a stroke, you'd see a fourth specialist. Elderly care thus tended to become seriously compartmentalized, with no single physician acting as quarterback, a situation that left many patients confused and dissatisfied.

Although the Royal College had supported my initiatives, the broader reception I received was neutral, at best. While physicians in Winnipeg and Halifax were sympathetic to my position, I was treated coolly in Vancouver and with some hostility in Toronto. In fact, at a meeting of several chiefs of medicine in Toronto to discuss these issues, one of them — he shall remain nameless — actually fell asleep. At another Toronto meeting, at Wellesley Hospital — it relied almost totally on subspecialties at the time — my pitch for a general internal medicine unit was dismissed. I maintained that if they continued on this path, residents would eventually choose to go elsewhere.

One prominent rheumatologist rose and declared that he disliked the tone of my speech because it implied that I was a better teacher than he was. And he'd been teaching for 40 years.

That wasn't remotely my intention, of course.

"I accept your opinion, sir," I said. "But I need to tell you that things have to change."

That exchange was typical of the battle I had to fight.

Wellesley Hospital did eventually change — but not fast enough. By the time it switched to a clinical teaching unit run by general internists, it was too late. In 2002, Wellesley effectively disappeared. Its teaching role was relinquished and its various departments were absorbed by St. Michael's Hospital.

It is not possible to draw a straight line between the renewed emphasis on general internal medicine and improved patient care. In fact, no study I am aware of has shown that changing the medical curriculum has bettered hospital results. Nevertheless, I'm convinced that this shift to new ideas did sharpen the skills of medical residents and lead to better job satisfaction. In turn, I would bet, that also led to improved patient care.

ON JULY 1, 1984, CANADA DAY, my family arrived in Toronto to begin the next chapter of our lives. For the previous 10 years, we had used the holiday to take the kids to a swimming pool or a park. On this occasion, I had an orientation day scheduled at the hospital. I set off cheerfully in the morning in my car and had not gone very far down Bathurst Street when I spotted a woman in a black cap trying to wave me down. Thinking she needed my help, I stopped.

It turned out she was a police officer, tagging me for speeding.

"But I was only going 60 kilometres an hour," I protested.

"The speed limit is 50," she said. "Oh, you have Quebec licence plates I see."

"Yes," I said, "the speed limit is 60 in Quebec, and I've just moved here, and it's my first day of work at the hospital. I'm on my way there now."

It was no use. She showed no mercy and promptly wrote up the ticket.

Welcome to Toronto, Dr. Ho Ping Kong.

TORONTO WESTERN, I FELT, WAS the right place for me. Its large downtown patient population, to which I was accustomed, meant that I would be faced with a goodly share of diagnostic challenges.

Not long after I began to practise there, I was reminded again how important it is during examinations, not only to look at the patient, but to see what you are looking at. In this instance, it wasn't my own powers of observation that mattered, but those of a sharp-eyed emergency ward nurse.

I was in the ER one afternoon when my resident, Dr. Jeannie Callum, presented a young woman named Emily, about 30 years old, who had been admitted with severe abdominal pain. Her blood pressure was normal but, while there was no specific mass detected, her abdomen was distended and there was marked tenderness. Then, while I was checking her, the nurse mentioned in passing that something strange had happened when the blood pressure reading had been taken. Emily's hand, involuntarily, had gone into spasm and formed itself into a cupped shape — a reaction medically known as carpopedal spasm (sometimes called Trousseau's sign or the obstetrician's hand).

I immediately turned to Dr. Callum and said, "I think your patient has acute pancreatitis."

"How do you know?"

I knew because, in patients with such conditions, it is not uncommon for the hand to go into spasm when the blood pressure cuff is applied. The precise physiology is complex: when you have pancreatitis, you release enzymes that lead to the formation of calcium deposits in the peritoneum, the lining of the abdominal cavity. In turn, serum calcium levels fall, sometimes precipitously. The low calcium (hypo-calcemia) causes spasm in the hand (carpopedal spasms). The hand then cups in the rough shape of an obstetrician delivering a baby. Some patients with low calcium levels also exhibit a facial tic known as Chvostek's sign; to detect it, the cheek is tapped gently with a finger over the facial nerve.

Our diagnosis was subsequently confirmed by a CT scan that revealed abdominal inflammation, and by high readings of the enzyme amylase in the blood. The treatment for this condition must be tailored to the specific situation, but in general it is important to rest the pancreas by not eating, and to administer calcium supplements to correct the deficit and eliminate the carpopedal spasms. Undiagnosed or unchecked, acute pancreatitis can lead to serious abdominal and lung problems.

There are, of course, dozens of names like Trousseau's sign and Chvostek's sign in the professional literature, usually named for the physicians that first discovered them (and sometimes for their patients). They tend to date from a period before the introduction of evidence-based medicine when experience and observation counted far more than science.

ANOTHER INTRIGUING CASE I RECALL involved a 30-year-old woman named Julia who had been referred to me with lumps on her Achilles tendons. She'd already had both a biopsy and an MRI, but no formal diagnosis. And she was clearly frustrated. When she initially appeared in my office, she refused to show me the lumps, explaining that she hated doctors. Finally prevailing upon her to let me examine one foot, I found lumps that were the size of small, two-inch potatoes. The second foot was the same. The nodules were large enough that Julia could wear only loose-fitting running shoes.

"I'll tell you what you have," I said. "You have tendinous xanthomatosis."

This is a rare, genetic condition under which lumps form on various parts of the body, including heels, elbows and knees. It is caused by an abnormality in the metabolism of cholesterol, which results in very high cholesterol readings. Hers was 10 (four is considered normal). Some forms of the disease are treatable by drugs. But Julia's form of the illness is more pernicious and less amenable to such therapy. I had to tell her that while we might be able to control the size of the nodules, we likely could not make them disappear. In the meantime, we also had to bring down her cholesterol levels, which would otherwise put her at risk for coronary heart disease and stroke.

I did, eventually, learn the source of Julia's animus against doctors. She was a single mother whose husband had died a few years earlier, at the age of 30, from pancreatic cancer. The tragedy had left her with bitter feelings for the medical profession. More than a decade later, I am still treating her, and I'm pleased to say she no longer holds us in contempt.

However, the larger lesson of this story is that a dozen fancy medical scans and even invasive tests were not required to diagnose the illness — only the powers of visual observation. That isn't always the case, of course. But it is the case more often than you might expect.

I was born in England and came to Canada at five. My dad was a cabinet maker. My mother worked for a cookie manufacturer. I have a high-school education and have worked ever since. I am 49. My illness just appeared, suddenly, without warning or known cause. I woke up one morning and had these lumps on the back of my feet. One was smaller than the other. That was about 13 years ago. No one else in the family has it.

I saw my family doctor, who said it was a result of wearing high heels. But I don't wear high heels. I didn't argue, but I knew that was wrong. I saw a second general practitioner who eventually sent me to Dr. Ho Ping Kong — HPK. I don't really mind doctors. I just like to joke around about it. But I was initially reluctant to show him the bumps, because it was embarrassing. Now, I'm okay with it. After looking at the lumps and feeling them, he told me I have a kind of xanthomatous. I went for various tests, a biopsy, an MRI, etc., which confirmed the diagnosis.

So it turns out there are two kinds of this illness and mine is the more serious type. It may take years to get better. It may not get better. It may get smaller or not. There is no pain, fortunately. I function and walk normally. It's just the visuals. I wear ankle boots in the winter, and Crocs in the summer. The bumps are just localized to this one area. I'm on Crestor for cholesterol, five milligrams per day. I take thyroid pills and have blood work done every three months. There are much worse things out there. So I accept it and I live with it. I can manage. It's part of my life. It seems to be working.

I see no other doctors. I'm comfortable with HPK. Some doctors don't sit and talk to you. Everybody's in a rush. But he isn't. We sit, we talk, we have a laugh. You should be able to do that. When I come here, I feel like I'm going to my second home. Doctors need to do that. They need to make the patient feel safe and comfortable.

NOT LONG AGO, A COLLEAGUE of mine, a rheumatologist, sent Evelyn to see me — a Chinese-Canadian medical research scientist in her mid-50s. Complaining of fatigue, she had been losing weight (about 20 pounds) and had developed tachycardia (a fast pulse), a tremor and a nagging cough. For the initial diagnosis, asthma, she'd been prescribed a puffer but, after a few weeks, it was clear this remedy was not working.

When Evelyn appeared in my office, her pulse rate was 140 beats per minute. I asked her to remove her sunglasses and, the moment she did, I was pretty sure I knew what was wrong with her.

"Tell me," I said, "are your eyes always like that?"

"Yes," she replied.

Her eyes were fixed and unblinking. In medical parlance, this was Stelwag's sign, a possible indicator of Graves' disease or hyperthyroidism. Its cause is essentially unknown, but it is likely an autoimmune disorder. And it is quite common in Asians, especially women. A familiar symptom of the ailment is bulging eyes, otherwise known as proptosis. The condition sensitizes human organs and tissue to adrenalin — the so-called fight-or-flight chemical.

On further examination, I found confirming evidence: an enlarged goitre — a swelling of the thyroid gland — and a thyroxine count near 100 (normal is 9–19 pmol/L). In fact, she was very close to thyroid storm, a potentially fatal event in which the thyroid gland suddenly releases large amounts of hormones.

It was 2005, the end of September, and I had just finished writing research grant proposals. My husband and I went fishing in the Thousand Islands. I developed a sore throat, came back and started coughing. This went on for a few months. The cough was so bad that, at times, I could not talk. My colleague suggested I see a respirologist. I was also losing weight, quite a lot of weight. I was happy having lost the weight but then, in one month, I lost 10 pounds. I now weighed less than 100 pounds, so I figured something was wrong. So instead of seeing the respirologist, I was referred to Dr. Ho Ping Kong. He was away on holiday and I remember a day where just crossing the street, I experienced severe shortness of breath.

So I went to a walk-in clinic. I suggested to the doctor there that it might be asthma. She listened to my lungs, but they were clear, so she gave me a puffer. I used it for a week without effect and finally went to see Ho Ping Kong. He took a full history, but his first question to me was "Are you nervous?" I said, "I know you are a big-shot doctor, but I am not intimidated." In fact, nervousness is one of the symptoms of this thyroid condition. So he hadn't even looked at my thyroid but he already knew. He told me right away what I had.

But I was surprised because in the year 2000, I'd had thyroid surgery to remove a cyst on one side. I'd lost half the thyroid. You wouldn't think half a thyroid could produce hyperthyroidism. It should have been hypo, not hyper, so it never crossed my mind. In fact, since I was a child, various doctors had looked at my eyes and suggested I might have a thyroid problem, but the tests had always come back normal. After a few more tests, he diagnosed Graves' disease, a form of hyperthyroidism. I took medication for about two years and I've been fine since then. I've been very privileged to have had him. As a medical researcher myself, it's hard for me to trust doctors. But that's not true of Dr. Ho Ping Kong.

HYPERTHYROIDISM IS OFTEN DIFFICULT TO diagnose because patients don't always exhibit the full range of symptoms. It might only be indicated by tachycardia or weight loss. For that reason, it is sometimes known as masked hyperthyroidism or apathetic hyperthyroidism.

In Evelyn's instance, everything pointed to the correct diagnosis, except her cough, which instinctively I ignored. But the other indicia (the fast pulse, weight loss, racial legacy and, most especially, fixed stare — what I saw when I looked directly at the patient) told me as much as I needed to know.

IT'S IMPORTANT TO MAKE CLEAR that no part of my argument should be interpreted as an indictment of medical technology. Quite the contrary. The truth is that many of the remarkable advances made in our understanding and treatment of disease would simply not have been possible without technological innovation. Technology has catalyzed less invasive surgical procedures, significantly reducing the length of hospital stays, rehabilitation times and costs. For tens of millions of ambulatory patients, a wide range of innovations — pacemakers, insulin pens, prosthetic devices, oxygen masks, to name a few — have greatly improved the quality of life.

In my own field, computed tomography (CT scans), magnetic image resonance (MRIs) and ultrasound imaging have made diagnosis of illness easier, faster and more precise.

For example, when I started practising in the 1960s, and for many years afterward, diagnosing something like a liver abscess was often difficult. Any number of conditions might have fit a patient presenting with fever and right-sided abdominal pain. Today, a single ultrasound or CT scan can make detecting that potentially fatal condition relatively easy.

In other instances, these scans can provide a critical complement to diagnoses made by the powers of human observation. In my early years in Toronto, I was sent a case involving Yolanda, a 40-year-old Guyanese woman suffering from sarcoidosis. One of many ailments still imperfectly understood, sarcoidosis is a multi-system disease characterized chiefly by inflammation, often of the lungs or lymph nodes. In some ways, the affected tissue resembles tuberculosis. Unlike TB, it is not infectious. It is, however, serious and can lead to serious complications, including respiratory failure and death, from involvement of the heart's electrical system.

Yolanda had already been diagnosed when she reported new and crippling pain in her hands. After she refused a bone biopsy recommended by a plastic surgeon, she was referred to me. I examined and felt her hands and immediately concluded she had sarcoidosis of the hands and bones. An MRI later verified that diagnosis.

Oddly enough, while I saw very little sarcoidosis in Jamaica, I saw it in England among Jamaicans who had moved to the U.K. — perhaps the result of living in a colder climate. The same later proved true in Toronto, among the expatriate Jamaican community. Fortunately, especially among young women, the ailment responds well to prednisone and is usually self-limiting. On the other hand, it can also affect the eyes, liver and the brain.

In Yolanda's case, it was the combination of physical diagnosis — seeing and feeling her hands — and the marvel of the MRI that allowed us to correctly identify her condition.

Of course, it is one thing to recognize a telltale symptom in a patient. It is another to know how to interpret it. On one occasion, a colleague of mine, an orthopedic surgeon, asked me to

THE ART OF MEDICINE

examine Nadia, a young woman of 29 years he suspected of having nephrotic syndrome — a kidney disorder. He was treating her because she had been born with what is known as a meningocele — a hernial protrusion of the meninges that damages the spinal cord. Despite her disability, she had been a talented wheelchair athlete in university and had found work after graduation in a bank. His diagnosis of nephrotic syndrome had been based on what appeared to be a solid clue — a sharp drop in protein (albumen) levels in Nadia's blood. When that happens, edema is often the result and, indeed, her legs were swollen.

When she came to see me, Nadia was wearing earrings. That might seem like an irrelevant detail. In fact, it is anything but. Her jewellery allowed me to see that her earlobes were moving involuntarily. That, in turn, immediately told me that something was wrong with her jugular venous pressure (JVP), one of the major clinical indices of heart failure. I suspected that her long years of enforced sitting had damaged her lungs, leading to right-sided heart failure, with incompetence in the heart's tricuspid valve.

Alternatively, I thought she might have cardiomyopathy, a disease of the heart muscle that causes edema and other serious problems. I was intuitively skeptical of the nephrotic syndrome diagnosis because her edema was largely confined to her legs, instead of where it usually is with this condition, in the face. I sent her to see a heart specialist (Dr. Tom Parker, who later became physician-in-chief at St. Michael's Hospital) who, after performing an angiogram and a cardiac biopsy, confirmed the cardiomyopathy, for which we treated her successfully.

Again, it was the mere sight of the involuntary earlobe fluctuations with each heartbeat that had pointed me in the right direction. When you see that, you know immediately that something serious is going on. Thus, while I never advise patients to wear earrings to appointments, I am never disappointed when they do. It certainly makes spotting anomalies in jugular venous pressure easier.

THE ART OF SEEING

NOT FAR FROM MY HOSPITAL office is a pharmacy I frequent. Over the years, I came to know its owners, an industrious couple from China. One day, I stopped in to pick up a prescription. When the owner approached the counter, I immediately noticed a lump in his neck.

"David," I said, "you have a small lump in your neck."

"Yes," he said, "I was planning to come and see you about it."

"What else is going on, medically?"

"A year ago, on a flight to Hong Kong, my nose became very stuffy and I had a nosebleed."

"Do you know what this is?"

He shook his head.

"It's probably nasopharyngeal carcinoma."

He came to my office the next day for an examination, a CT scan and a biopsy, which confirmed my instinct.

How could I make the diagnosis so quickly, on the evidence of only a lump and a nosebleed? I knew that David was in a vulnerable category. South Chinese men and women in their 40s are the prime victims of the disease. My own father had been diagnosed with it, also in his 40s, and been successfully cured with radiation. David's case was more advanced and he thus underwent both radiation and chemotherapy, and four years later he seems to be cured.

Sensitive clinicians, however, will not only rely on their eyes to make a diagnosis. As we will see in the next chapters, they will also learn to use the extraordinary powers of the human ear and of human touch.

Dr. RODRIGO CAVALCANTI

Dr. Rodrigo Cavalcanti is program director for the General Internal Medicine Subspecialty Training Program at the University Toronto and director of scholarship at the Centre for Excellence in Education and Practice (CEEP). An assistant professor of medicine at the University of Toronto, he holds an M.D. degree and an M.Sc. degree in clinical epidemiology, both from the University of Toronto, and a diploma in tropical medicine from the Gorgas Course (University of Alabama and Universidad Peruana Cayetano Heredia).

THE OFFSPRING OF A QUÉBÉCOIS mother and a Brazilian father, Dr. Rodrigo Cavalcanti developed an interest in biology as a youth and was initially torn between studying plant or molecular biology. In time, however, he found pure science unsatisfying, because it lacked the human element. "Medicine," he says, "was biology with a human interaction." Drawn at first to neurology, he ultimately concluded that, too often, once the diagnosis was made, there "was not a lot to offer the patient. And I enjoyed the diagnostic process which is central to internal medicine."

He was first exposed to Dr. Herbert Ho Ping Kong as a second-year resident, in 1998. "His reputation preceded him," Cavalcanti says. "He uses the Socratic method, asking questions that make you think, not the standard questions, but questions that force you to think laterally. I was impressed not only by his knowledge, but by his ability to connect with patients — with everyone really — on a human level and to prioritizing that connection."

Cavalcanti maintains that the long, three-decade run of hard, science-driven, evidence-based practice has reached the end of its course, as a paradigm. Increasingly, he says, organized medicine is recognizing the signal importance of the art of medicine, "the need to make a connection between two human beings, the healer and the patient." In fact, he points out, that art was originally embedded in the core elements of the evidence-based model.

"I like to remind people that its fundamental tenets were to make decisions informed by evidence, to interpret the quality of the evidence, and a third principle, which people forget, of incorporating patient preference." The original intent, which grew out of the work of David Sackett and others, was to have that conversation. "Research and statistics gives you a good idea about what the average experience will be," Cavalcanti says. "But the uncertainty will be greatest at the individual level. Even if you had perfect evidence, you have to make judgment calls."

The human factor became diminished, however, as physicians wrestled with the massive gaps in the quality of the scientific evidence. Most of the profession's energies were directed toward filling those gaps.

Among Cavalcanti's current research interests is the Grey Zone of diagnostic medicine. "We conceptualize diagnosis as firm, rule-based clear-boundary categories," he says. "But the reality is they are somewhat artificial labels that we assign to these biologic phenomena. Experienced clinicians get that. They've seen enough to know the label covers a large variation."

Recently, for example, a middle-aged woman presented with liver disease. Certain signs pointed to Budd-Chiari syndrome, a rare condition caused by hepatic blood clots. But other variables, including liver enzyme levels, did not fit the disease at all. In that situation, he says, you either need the clinical experience or a healthy dose of skepticism to challenge the weight of evidence. In the end, the patient turned out to have partial Budd-Chiari.

"So you have two Grey Zones, effectively," Cavalcanti observes. "The first is what is the proper label to attach to this condition? And then you have the suspicion of a clear label, but doubt and uncertainty. Western medicine is built on the foundation of diagnosis informing prognosis and treatment. But sometimes there is no clear diagnosis, just a patient with symptoms and a need for care. That's the art of medicine, recognizing that the ultimate purpose of medicine is to comfort and treat and help them cope with their experience. It's managing uncertainty because you won't always get the answer. In that situation, you devise a plan of action that seems reasonable, but you must come clean about the limits of knowledge and where your thinking is going. I tell patients, 'Here's what we know and here's what we don't know and here's where we can possibly go together.'"

Many young medical students, he concedes, are more interested in acquiring raw medical knowledge than in the niceties and nuances of the bedside art. "The science is important, but I think educators need to communicate that there's more to it than that, and communicate it early on."

Cavalcanti says he detects among the newer generation of graduates a shift away from the embrace of medical science as the only thing. Part of that is the result of choosing more well-rounded candidates for med school. Narrative medicine — recognition that the patient's personal story carries as much weight as the more objective classification and recommendation for treatment — is also gaining traction in a few major American medical schools, but, he adds, "I think there's still a lot to be done."

During patient encounters, many students are so preoccupied with remembering everything they are supposed to remember that they have trouble being open about what they don't know. "And the amount of information is so overwhelming, it's easy to default on thinking on the knowledge side of things."

And although modern technology has made medical information more readily accessible, so that it may no longer be necessary to have to retain it all, the reality is that "you still have to internalize and organize that knowledge," he says. Exams usually have right or wrong answers. In the real world of medicine, Cavalcanti says, patients are more complicated. "There, the challenge is to apply your knowledge in search of the best answer and to acquire more knowledge. For example, if you find fluid in the patient's abdomen, you need to know where else to look. I have to know what I know in order to ask the right questions."

Even then, because any specific piece of information likely has at least a degree of uncertainty, "You need to be able to integrate your other knowledge to help make the diagnosis," Cavalcanti says.

Perceiving "what is really there" is an art best developed over time. "It takes years. When I teach students how to palpate the heart, I tell them, 'This is a marathon. It will take you four years or longer to learn to do this properly. Today is the first step in the marathon.'"

Dr. PETER SINGER

Peter Singer studied internal medicine at University of Toronto, medical ethics at University of Chicago, public health at Yale University and management at Harvard Business School. Since May 2010, he has been CEO of Grand Challenges Canada, a federally funded project aimed at improving lives in low- and middle-income societies through integrative scientific, health-related and business initiatives. A director at the Sandra Rotman Centre, University Health Network and University of Toronto, Singer — an Order of Canada recipient — is also a professor of medicine at University of Toronto, and the foreign secretary of the Canadian Academy of Health Science. He has served as an adviser to the Bill & Melinda Gates Foundation, the U.N. Secretary General's office, the government of Canada, BioVeda China Fund and several African governments on global health. With Dr. Abdallah Daar, he co-authored The Grandest Challenge: Taking Life-Saving Science from Lab to Village.

PETER SINGER'S INTEREST IN MEDICAL ETHICS — and ethics as a portal into the art of medicine — began in high school, in the late 1970s. Long before bioethics was even a blip on the profession's radar screen, a grade 13 biology teacher assigned him a paper on the ethics of human subjects research. It immediately galvanized his interest. But his real epiphany came during his years as an intern at Toronto Western Hospital.

"I was caring for a patient on the hematology ward and she had widespread cervical cancer and was dying," he recalls. "And I came to realize that, while we could rattle off 15 causes why her potassium or phosphorus levels were low or high, when it came time to decide whether we would resuscitate her, we would scribble it in pencil on the nursing notes and then rub it out afterwards. There was no honest conversation, either with her or her family or among the staff. I thought we could bring more rigour to that kind of situation."

Among his most memorable teachers at Western was Herbert Ho Ping Kong. HPK was considered a paradigm of the old school master of the art of medicine, "both in the way he taught students, at the bedside and on rounds, and in respect to physical exam. Herbert was particularly good at elements of problem solving, taking cognate factoids and turning them into a diagnosis and plan, the judgmental part. There was a lot of lateral thinking. He would always examine things no one else would examine, such as the Sister Mary Joseph's Nodule, a lymph node close to the belly button that, when bulging, may be a sentinel of abdominal cancer. Or he'd always be listening for abdominal bruits, which no one else did."

In a more formal classroom setting, to test the class's knowledge of symptoms, HPK would demonstrate a patient's gait, or ask a student to emulate it, making education more interactive. A favoured gambit was a form of paraphasia, in which he would "say something seemingly irrelevant or tangential. It might be drawn from the day's weather forecast or from a current event and, by the end of the process, the search for the diagnosis of the case under discussion, you'd understand that he had provided a clue to the right answer." Some of that, Singer suspects, was derived from HPK's Jesuitical training and thinking. And his playfulness, he adds, may have spring from the *joie de vivre* embedded in Jamaica's cultural context.

In general, Ho Ping Kong was, for Singer, a major resource for the less common illnesses and syndromes. "He wasn't the evidence based person who covered the more common things you saw 90 percent of the time; he was the guy who covered the thousand things you might see 10 percent of the time, the rare and the exotic — dengue or break-bone fever, porphyrias, malaria."

Singer's work ultimately went a different direction — bioethics.

What is framed at the surface of the ethics issue, he says, has a lot to do with the prevailing narrative of people's lives. "An individual's previous contextualized narrative experiences influences a lot of their responses to health care situations."

The art of medicine is a term that encompasses a broad range of professional skills — from taking the patient's history and conducting the physical exam, to the bedside diagnosis and plan of action, to the broader sense of caring. One of the best quotes on the subject, Singer suggests, is American clinician Francis Peabody's dictum, "The secret of the care of the patient is in caring for the patient."

Peabody's full quote, from a 1927 paper, provides a deeper context.

Disease in man is never exactly the same as disease in an experimental animal, for in man the disease at once affects and is affected by what we call the emotional life. Thus, the physician who attempts to take care of a patient while he neglects this factor is as unscientific as the investigator who neglects to control all the conditions that may affect his experiment. The good physician knows his patients through and through, and his knowledge is bought dearly. Time, sympathy and understanding must be lavishly dispensed, but the reward is to be found in that personal bond which forms the greatest satisfaction of the practice of medicine. One of the essential qualities of the clinician is interest in humanity, for the secret of the care of the patient is caring for the patient.

SINGER ALSO CITES A LANDMARK 1978 journal article by American bioethicist Edmund Pellegrino on "Ethics and the Moment of Clinical Truth" — the moment being that point at which the physician must make a clinical decision and choose what should be done from the menu of things that could be done.

After earning his medical degree in Toronto, Singer studied under two giants in the field, Mark Siegler, director of the University of Chicago's MacLean Center for Clinical Medical Ethics, and with Alvan Feinstein at Yale. In one journal article, Siegler argued that the art of medicine requires knowledge of many ethical issues, including informed consent, truth-telling, confidentiality, end-of-life care, pain relief and patient rights. "Medicine, even at its most technical and scientific," he wrote, "is an encounter between human beings, and the physician's work of diagnosing disease, offering advice and providing treatment is embedded in a moral context."

Feinstein, in his work on clinimetrics, maintained that medicine had become too hardened and too scientific. Blood potassium levels, to cite one example, were much easier to measure than the degree of pain. That professional bias, Singer contends — the dominance of hard-side data over soft — is at least as true today as it was when Feinstein wrote, or when Abraham Flexner published his groundbreaking report on medical education in America in 1910.

But the art of medicine isn't only about Big Think moral issues. Sometimes, Singer says, it's about what might otherwise seem to be the most inconsequential aspects of practice. "A doctor enters a hospital room to take a patient's blood pressure and other readings. The patient, in bed, is thirsty, and there's a beaker of water and an empty glass on the portable bed table. But he can't reach it or pour it himself. Well, the art of medicine here is taking the beaker and filling the glass and handing it to the patient, even if you are there to do something else. It sounds trivial, but is actually archetypal."

In terms of end-of-life care, he says, "It really came down to three questions to be asked at the bedside. Is the patient in pain or experiencing other symptoms? Have they prepared with family for the end of life? And are there wishes regarding life-sustaining treatment known?"

Singer believes that the easier part of these skills — more effective communication and sensitivity — can and are being taught to medical students. "The harder part is teaching leadership and judgment. That too can be taught but to what degree?" Empathy is an important factor: "The ability to put oneself in the shoes of the patient, separated from family and children, dealing with disease and death, and translating that empathy into a higher standard of care."

Does the art of medicine apply to Singer's current work in social innovation? He's convinced that it does. By the summer of 2013, his Grand Challenges Canada had funded 400 separate projects, many of them just beginning to deliver results. One of them involved working with an NGO in Nigeria around women's and children's health issues. Traditionally, he says, the messages delivered at Friday sermons in mosques implicitly or explicitly discouraged women from seeking medical care for themselves and their children. The NGO intervention is aimed at using more educated imams to teach conservative imams about the importance of vaccination and other aspects of neonatal care. The evaluations so far are encouraging.

More broadly, it is clear that the same questions that determine attendance at health clinics in the developed world — do women feel safe and comfortable? — are critical determinants of attendance in the developing world as well. "It's exactly what you would expect," Singer says, "but we tend not to think about the interpersonal aspects of care. And they are critical, because the goal is to encourage women to come to these facilities for care. And they need to feel comfortable." Some of this, he says, is the result of "the callousness of physicians and other health workers, mistreating women, often poorer women." Cultural mores are "hard to change quickly, but they can be changed with time."

CHAPTER 5

The ART
of LISTENING

Listen to your patient.
He is telling you the diagnosis.
— Sir William Osler

SEVERAL YEARS AGO, A CHINESE-CANADIAN named Charles developed a nagging pain in his back. He was about 56 years old and, though he had prospered since he'd immigrated, and managed to save enough funds to own a building, he continued to work as a labourer, loading boxes of vegetables on and off delivery trucks. He continued to work through the pain for about a month but, eventually, it grew so severe that he had to stop. Through his employer, Charles consulted an orthopedic specialist retained by the Workers' Compensation Board. The doctor diagnosed osteoarthritis and prescribed painkillers.

But by then, Charles had also started to lose weight. He was sent for a series of tests, which indicated the presence of red blood cells in his urine. That finding raised the possibility of kidney disease, so he was sent to a nephrologist who did further tests, confirming that Charles's urine contained blood, and suggested that he might have IgA (immunoglobulin A) nephropathy, a common kidney disease that affects the organ's filters, or glomeruli. Although the condition is mostly benign, the kidney may, over time, lose its ability to cleanse the blood properly.

However, just as a precaution, he also decided to test for bladder cancer. So Charles was sent to his third specialist, a urologist, where he underwent a cystoscopy, a procedure that provides a better view of tumours or stones. The test came back negative, which appeared to reconfirm the original diagnosis of IgA nephropathy.

With that, the medical system was largely done with Charles. His family physician prescribed analgesics for the continuing back pain, but was otherwise at a loss to explain what exactly was going on. Unfortunately, the pain was getting worse and Charles had become virtually incapacitated. By the sixth month of his illness, sick and continuing to lose weight (about 30 pounds in total), he could hardly walk.

At that point the family doctor referred him to me. When Charles appeared with his wife in my office for the first time, he almost had to crawl into the room.

"Dr. Ho Ping Kong," he pleaded, "you have to do something. Otherwise, I'm going to die."

"Don't worry," I said, though I really had no reason to offer this assurance. "We will figure out what's wrong with you."

He sat down and began to recount his medical history.

Then, because I do it almost instinctively, I decided to start the physical examination by listening to his heart. What I heard, immediately, was the signature *whoosh, whoosh* of a systolic murmur, a five on a scale of six at his apex.

"I know what's wrong with you," I said. "You have subacute endocarditis" (an infection in the heart valve).

This diagnosis was confirmed by details provided by further examination — clubbing of his fingers and the temporary blackening of his little finger, a few weeks earlier.

Charles was admitted to hospital and, within 24 hours, a

cardiac surgeon installed a pacemaker and replaced the diseased mitral valve with a mechanical one. The infection itself was treated successfully with antibiotics. Today, Charles functions at about 85 or 90 percent of what might be considered normal. In another month, without intervention, he would likely have died. His life was literally saved by the simple act of listening.

Instinctively, I had a sense that endocarditis might be at work. It was suggested by the combination of symptoms — excruciating backache, weight loss and blood in the urine. But his case also speaks to the compartmentalization that has come to characterize modern medical practice. Expertise is acquired in subspecialties, and that expertise is invaluable. But physicians often lose the ability to focus on the big picture.

A PATIENT'S TESTIMONY — *Charles M.* ——————————

I was born in 1953 in a small village on mainland China. I came to Canada at 23, in 1977, after two months in Hong Kong. It was very bad time in China, for virtually everybody. Everyone wanted to leave the Communist system. You could not own your own house or car or business and you could not have independent ideas. You were forbidden to listen to outside radio or read foreign newspapers. It's better today, but still quite restrictive.

I had been a student. I came to Toronto and worked in a furniture-assembly factory, but not for long. I quit the job because I was using a spray gun to paint the furniture and it made me sick. Then the government of Canada gave me money to study English. I set up a factory to manufacture tofu for restaurants and supermarkets, which I eventually sold, after 16 years, to my brothers. When I sold it, it was grossing $1.5 million in revenue. That's a lot of tofu.

I became sick in May 2007 after coming back from

China. I was nauseous. I was very tired and did not want to eat food. In June, I started getting intense lower back pain. I could not stand or walk. I was working in a clothing factory, as a labourer, but had to quit because of the pain. I went to see my family doctor who sent me to the hospital. They checked my kidneys, but it was normal. Then they checked my lungs because I was having trouble breathing, but they were normal. I went to three separate hospitals and had no answer. So I went to see another family doctor and he sent me to Ho Ping Kong.

I was so sick. I was losing weight. I thought I would die. I could not sleep or walk. Painkillers helped, but only for a few hours. I was very lucky. Ho Ping Kong saw me the next day. I was late for the appointment and I worried that he'd have left. But he waited. My wife brought me. I was in a wheelchair. Parts of my body had turned black and swollen. My fingers, the soles of my feet. It was bacteria in my blood. He asked me very detailed but clear questions. I was with him an hour. I was admitted for two weeks. I was very sick. I was scared because I knew something serious was wrong. So they eventually confirmed the doctor's diagnosis, but they also had to repair the valve, which the bacteria had eaten away. So I had the surgery and since then I feel better, normal. My appetite returned. So I am very grateful. Now I walk two hours every day, but slowly, because otherwise my heart goes too fast. Dr. Ho Ping Kong has helped me with everything, even with helping me fill out forms for social security. We are all very lucky to be in Canada. It gave us a chance. It saved us.

CHARLES'S CASE ALSO UNDERSCORED THE signal importance of listening to the heart. Not long ago, Toronto Western Hospital played host to Dr. Rory McCallum, a promising Irish nephrologist who was here as a visiting clinical fellow and is now on staff. He expressed an interest in medical education, so I introduced him to Harvey, our high-tech cardio-pulmonary simulator. We use it to teach some 25 separate cardiac functions, including blood pressure, heart sounds and a variety of heart murmurs. In about 10 minutes, I showed him four different murmurs.

Afterward, in a little test, he was able to correctly identify two out of the four. He was not terribly happy with the result, but the very next week, he was doing rounds at the Toronto General Hospital when he met a patient suspected of having IgA nephropathy, because of red blood cells in the urine. What did he do? He immediately put the stethoscope on the patient's heart and heard the systolic murmur and said to his startled residents, "Change the diagnosis. This man has endocarditis."

At the centre of the art of listening lies the humble stethoscope. Invented by René Laennec in Paris in 1816, its first incarnation was scarcely more than a wooden tube. It functioned much like the ear trumpet, a device that augmented sound for the hearing impaired. Another 35 years passed before the first binaural stethoscope appeared, invented by Irishman Arthur Leared. The design of the modern instrument was established in the early 1850s as well, although a variety of technical improvements have naturally been made.

The stethoscope — from the Greek words *stethos* for chest, and *scopos* for examination — puts an educated ear to several key organs: the heart, lungs, abdomen, intestines, even specific veins and arteries. In tandem with the sphygmomanometer, it is also used in one of the most essential medical readings — blood pressure.

During my training in Jamaica, where we used murmurs to diagnose dozens of cases of rheumatic heart disease, the stethoscope was an invaluable tool. Patients encouraged us to use the device, which they called a trumpet. "Doctor," they would say, "you haven't yet sounded me with the trumpet." No visit was complete without that procedure. For them, it was viewed not only a method of diagnosis, but as a form of therapy.

But as my Toronto Western Hospital colleague Dr. Lisa Richardson has observed, the stethoscope is more than it might seem. It also serves to forge a connection between doctor and patient. It's more than a symbolic link. Active listening signals to patients that you care about them and are willing to take the time to listen to their organs. The judgment works the other way as well. If you don't use the stethoscope, it tells the patient that you are too busy or simply don't care enough to listen, an interpretation that will do nothing to nurture trust.

This is not a trivial issue. With the exponential increase in medical malpractice suits, physicians have lost the high level of trust they were once accorded almost automatically. Now, we are just as likely to be regarded with caution, wariness, even suspicion. Increasingly, patients are on the alert. A surgeon with a 95 percent success rate in the operating room may be entitled to respect, but the rest of us must earn it, every day.

Trust, rapport, communication — by any name, it's a critical component of the art of medicine. Various studies, in fact, have demonstrated that a high percentage of lawsuits result from a simple failure to communicate with patients.

So how do you encourage a patient to trust you? The answer may be as simple as eye contact. Far too many doctors spend too much time looking everywhere but at the patient. They are glancing at the desktop computer or reading the patient's file, but seldom actively engaging with the other person in the room, eye to eye. I once treated a British-Jamaican woman who insisted on coming back to see me in preference to her own family doctor. When I asked her why, she said, "Because you always look me in the eye."

When I first meet a new patient, I often ask questions that have no apparent connection to the matter at hand, the illness or problem that brought them to me. Where were you born?

THE ART OF LISTENING

What kind of work do you do? Tell me about your family. Simple questions, unlikely to tell me anything useful for diagnosis, but invaluable for establishing a solid foundation for the doctor-patient relationship. Such inquiries signal to the patient that he or she is not simply a disease or a syndrome, but a human being.

Occasionally, it is true, I will encounter a patient that resents such questions. An immigrant, for example, may interpret the question, "Where are you from?" as suggesting that he or she is not truly a Canadian. Others may feel that such information is none of my business. But in most instances, such questions help "break the ice" and facilitate the building of trust.

Particularly in the grey areas of medicine, where neither surgery nor pharmacopeia can cure disease, trust is vitally important. To some extent, trust by itself can be a kind of healer, assuring the patient that he or she has not been forgotten by the system, that everything that can possibly be done is being done, that someone in authority actually cares.

AT TIMES, IT'S A COMBINATION of listening and visual observation that proves diagnostically decisive. I recall seeing Brenda, a 50-year-old Jewish woman from Cape Town, South Africa, suffering from what is known as arteriovenous malformation (AVM) — a hereditary condition that makes a jumble of the body's arteries and veins.

AVMs can occur anywhere in the body, but they are particularly challenging when they appear in the brain. There, they behave like space-occupying lesions, producing (depending on the severity) headache, epilepsy, vertigo, muscle weakness, problems with balance and coordination and, most worrisomely, bleeding. The latter development can be catastrophic.

Brenda had already been to see a colleague of mine, Dr. Karel Terbrugge, an interventional neuro-radiologist. He'd successfully performed embolic therapy, with glass beads or glue to prevent bleeding, a very delicate procedure. A cavernous AVM is a significant medical problem. It wasn't that long ago that we had no good treatment for this condition.

When I finally met Brenda, she told me that, some 20 years earlier, she had been treated at Cape Town's prestigious Groote Schuur Hospital. That, of course, is where the late Christiaan Barnard performed the world's first successful heart transplant surgery, in 1967. There, Brenda had been diagnosed with Takayasu's disease, a form of giant-cell arteritis. A disease of the aorta, it generally affects young or middle-aged women, mostly of Asian origin. In my career, I had encountered it once or twice. It seemed unlikely that a Jewish woman from South Africa would have an Asian disease, but who was I to argue with the Groote Schuur Hospital?

I began to examine her and put my stethoscope on the skull. Instantly, I detected the bruit or vascular murmur. I could literally hear her AV malformation, even through the skull. But what was causing it?

I asked her to flex the joints of her thumb. To my surprise, she was able to bend it backwards almost 180 degrees. This, I knew, was a distinguishing feature of Ehlers-Danlos syndrome, a relatively uncommon connective tissue disorder named for a Danish and a French physician respectively. The disease manifests itself in various ways, including both hyper-flexibility of joints (the result of defects in the connective tissue) and blood vessel disorders that may lead to AV malformation.

Brenda had waited 20 years for the correct diagnosis. We were able to manage the illness for about a decade, but its progress is inexorable. Eventually, the blood vessels ruptured, causing internal bleeding and a lethal stroke.

WHEN WE SPEAK ABOUT THE art of listening, I am generally referring to the use of the stethoscope to hear heart murmurs or bruits indicative of other diseases. But listening to the patient can also mean something else — actually hearing what he or she tells you. Some time ago, a colleague asked me to see the husband of one of his attending staff. Fred, 49, was a grain broker who'd been ill for six months, suffering from anemia and an enlarged spleen. He was awaiting an appointment with a hematologist. I agreed to call him, not sure what exactly I'd be able to do.

After the telephone preliminaries, I started asking questions. "What seems to be the problem?"

"Well, doctor, I'm sweating at nights and have lost about 10 pounds and may have a slight fever. I'm not sure."

"Have you been sick before?"

"Never."

"Well, I'll try and see you in the next few days, but maybe I can speed things up by asking a few more questions. You're sure you've never been sick?"

"I've never been sick," Fred insisted. "I only have a mitral valve prolapse. I've had it for 20 years."

MVP occurs when the valve between the heart's left atrium and left ventricle fails to close properly, which can lead to leakage. At any time, about 15 percent of the population walks around with this condition, usually without any problems.

"Are you on medication for it?"

"No."

"Do you have a heart murmur?"

"Yes, doctor. I've also had a murmur for the last 20 years."

Bingo. "Listen, go the lab now and have some blood cultures done. Come and see me tomorrow. I think I know what's wrong with you."

Examining him the next day, I found both the enlarged spleen and a subconjunctival hemorrhage and heard his murmur, quite distinct, a five on a scale of six. The blood work further indicated that he was slightly anemic, had an elevated sedimentation rate (suggesting inflammation), tested positive for rheumatoid factor, had red blood cells in his urine and was growing a strain of streptococcus bug.

"You have endocarditis, and you have to be admitted to hospital immediately."

"I need to pick up my kids," he protested.

"You'll have to find someone else. I want you to go straight to Toronto General."

We started treating him with antibiotics and he responded well. One day, however, driving home from work, Fred developed dizziness and a cerebral embolus, a legacy of his heart valve problem. After a confirming MRI, we decided to replace the valve. At the time there were two choices, a pig valve, which lasts 10 years, or a mechanical valve, which lasts 20 years. The latter option, however, requires anticoagulation drugs. An active skier, Fred opted for the pig valve. But he was lucky enough to end up in the hands of Toronto General Hospital cardiac surgeon Tirone David, who managed to repair the original valve.

Twelve years later, Fred is thriving.

ONE DAY, DENISE, A 32-YEAR-OLD woman, came to visit me, complaining of high blood pressure. A civil servant, she had a high-stress job that might have been to blame, managing more than 1,000 people. Feeling unwell, she had paid a visit to a walk-in clinic. Her blood pressure was measured at 190/90 and she was prescribed blood pressure medication. The drug helped, reducing her blood pressure to 160/90, but she still felt stressed. I saw her a few weeks later.

Her history revealed no sweating or palpitations. Apart from the elevated blood pressure, she was a healthy young woman. I then looked for secondary evidence, given her relatively young

THE ART OF LISTENING

age. I put my trusted stethoscope to her right kidney and immediately heard it — a distinct bruit, as loud as I had ever heard, a six on a scale of six. I immediately rounded up some students to listen to it as well. Normally, the sound you hear has a clear to-and-fro quality. In Denise, there was no such flow, just a consistent one-way, systolic sound.

The bruit was an unmistakable sign of renal artery stenosis, a narrowing of blood flow to this vital organ. Because of it, the body's hormonal equilibrium had been upset, yielding hypertension. Fortunately, we had discovered the problem at an early stage, which enabled us to insert a surgical stent to open the artery and restore proper blood flow. Ten years later, Denise requires only a small amount of medication to control her blood pressure, and has experienced no further problems.

SOMETIMES, THE ART OF LISTENING can be used to integrate other clinical evidence and come to a more precise diagnosis. On one occasion, I led a group of medical students to examine Felix, a 50-year-old Portuguese man diagnosed the previous night with deep vein thrombosis, a blood clot in his leg. He was already taking heparin, a blood thinner, to prevent further clotting.

"Feel the leg," I instructed one of the residents. "How does it feel?"

"Cold," he said.

"And if you have a deep vein thrombosis, it should be . . . what?"

"Warm," he said.

"Correct . . . Therefore, this is not a deep vein thrombosis. So what is it? Look at his head. What do you see?"

"It's moving," another resident said.

"And that is known as . . . ?"

"The head nodding sign."

"Correct."

Formally known as de Musset's sign — after French poet and dramatist Alfred de Musset, who died at age 47 of heart failure — the head nodding sign is an indication of aortic insufficiency, typically involving a valve malfunction. The head bobs involuntarily in tandem with the beating of the heart.

We took Felix's blood pressure, which was 140/50.

"What does that tell us?" I asked.

"His pulse is collapsing," offered one of the students.

"Correct. So we have a cold leg, a collapsing pulse and the head nodding sign. Which means there's a leak somewhere, and we should be able to hear it."

Sure enough, when we listened to his heart, we heard the distinct *whoosh, whoosh* of a murmur, over the aortic valve.

The residents then took turns listening to the murmur.

Then I pressed the stethoscope onto Felix's femoral artery. Here, too, we could detect an audible diastolic murmur. This is Duroziez's sign, another indicator of aortic insufficiency. It is named for 19th-century French physician Paul Louis Duroziez, a pioneer in cardiac medicine.

"So this patient," I said, "unfortunately has endocarditis. His temperature was as high as 102 degrees. So why is the leg cold? It should be warm."

The students weren't sure.

Then one of the senior residents offered the right explanation. "Part of the vegetation on the aortic valve broke off and went to his leg. It has embolized and is thus blocking the flow of blood."

"That's correct," I said. "The likely culprit is a bacteria like staphylococcus aureus."

We immediately changed the diagnosis, from deep vein thrombosis to septic embolism, and began administering antibiotics for the endocarditis.

The next day, surgeon Dr. Tirone David replaced his infected aortic valve and, in the process, invented a new procedure to treat his septal abscess. We were unable to save Felix's leg — the infection had progressed too far — but we saved his life with the surgery and the antibiotics.

For me, this case represents the critical importance not only of listening and palpating, but of then integrating the knowledge gleaned to reach the diagnosis.

Dr. DANIEL PANISKO

Dr. Daniel Panisko is director of the undergraduate Medical Education Program, University of Toronto; a professor of Medicine at the University of Toronto; a member of the Clinical Studies Resource Centre at the Toronto Western Research Institute and director of the Master Teacher Program, for faculty and senior trainees.

DR. DANIEL PANISKO GREW UP in North Winnipeg, the son of a mechanical engineer (father) and a bookkeeper. Fascinated by sciences and stories of medical discovery, medicine was a natural attraction. By 23, he was a graduate doctor from the University of Manitoba. "Was that too young?" he asks. "It wasn't for me. I was pretty sure what I wanted career-wise. But it might be for some people. Some people might need and want more time and exposure to a broader range of experience."

He completed his core residency in Toronto and specialized in tropical medicine. Near the end of his course work, on a flight to a conference in Washington, D.C., he bumped into his old University of Toronto teacher, Dr. Herbert Ho Ping Kong.

"He asked me what I was doing the next year and I said I did not know," Panisko recalls. "It turned out Herbert had an opening for a clinical associate in internal medicine."

Panisko seized the opportunity and for the next three years immersed himself in patient care. He spent another year earning a master's of Public Health at Johns Hopkins. "I knew I wasn't going to be a researcher. Part of my attraction to medicine has always been the desire to work with people. I didn't want to spend 80 percent of my time in the lab or doing stats."

If art is an expression of man's humanity, Panisko says, then the art of medicine is what is human about medicine. "It takes several forms. There's the compassion part — the face-to-face contact and empathy. There's the creativity part — problem-solving in medicine, and in the health care system, because finding solutions for patients often does not follow a prescribed pattern. And there is the thinking outside the box part, being ready for differences, individualities, nuances. The science of medicine is protocolized. 'Here is the route and this is what you will follow.' Too many people are being railroaded into that box. The art lies in dealing with the patient who may not fit into that box. How do you decide if he does or doesn't? How do you accommodate them and not get frustrated, but learn to enjoy those differences and diversity?"

Although some observers believe the great pendular shift to the science side of the equation has begun to tilt back, Panisko isn't persuaded. The economics of modern medicine, he says, create severe time pressures — pressures for efficiencies. The system is built on a foundation of "volume-funded care and pushing patients through too fast, without time for personal reflection, without time for the patient."

Doctors are responding to the growing waiting lists and the shortage of family physicians. But they are also motivated, he says, by the desire to earn triple-digit salaries. "You hear about clinics that will only schedule one doctor on overnight call. They don't want to bring in additional staff because it will split the revenue stream. It would be saner and healthier and more humanistic for patients, but it isn't happening."

The medical community, he says, is also wrestling with the question of whether the new generation of doctors is — or may become — too reliant on technology, at the expense of humanism. "It's a huge debate, particularly in medical education. Are we all going to become cyborgs, perpetually attached to devices of some kind? Or do we take advantage of technology to accelerate and magnify what we can do — so it becomes power? Technology, we know, is fallible."

Still, Panisko thinks younger doctors are at once more conversant with and more dependent on technology. It's a trend he expects to increase, because it "does yield efficiencies and it does help doctors deal with the vast amounts of new information. But this does not diminish the importance of the art of medicine."

Medical educators are also pondering how much students actually need to learn, given the exponential growth of information. "There are more diseases, more drugs, and therefore more side effects," Panisko says. "And we understand mechanisms more. But what proportion do we need to know? Arguably, training would be better aimed at teaching problem-solving techniques, including how to search and find relevant information at point of care. It's constantly evolving."

Other aspects of medical education are also evolving, including how to combat the erosion of ethics and empathy that has historically marked the passage of students through med school. New studies, Panisko says, suggest that a direct apprenticeship system and a "longitudinal relationship" with a single physician/ role model confers a better understanding of what proper treatment should be.

Imagine, he says, that you are an overworked medical student on a late-night round in the emergency department. Your default-setting attitude is slightly negative or frustrated. A patient is admitted with an overdose of some kind. Your reflex tendency will be to blame the patient for his or her social behaviour. That is roughly how the current system works — encounters with patients are episodic.

In the longitudinal model, originated at the University of Minnesota in the 1970s and now in place, in whole or in part, at 11 of 17 Canadian medical schools, students work with a single doctor for three or six months and get to know patients in a more complete way. So when a patient arrives in emergency at 3 a.m. in crisis, "you know his or her background and the whole person."

Research at Harvard University suggests that this approach

— more contact with the patient, more contact with the supervisor/teacher — reduces the degree of ethical erosion in new doctors. "The other system," says Panisko, in which you bounce from one preceptor to another, and one rotation to the next, always encountering new challenges and affronts to the ego because of what you do not know, induces "a certain hardening. In the longitudinal relationship, there's more mentorship. The student is less likely to get lost in the shuffle. You can see if the student is feeling down or needs help." The University of Toronto is hoping to pilot its version of this curriculum approach in 2014 or 2015.

Panisko sees a generational shift in the doctors coming up through the system — more interest in quality-of-life issues (hours of work per week), the extent to which medical training will impinge on personal lives and remuneration. "That's new," he says. "Those questions never came up when I trained. Now they are top of mind."

The other reality is that the market for some high-priced medical specialties is now saturated. In Toronto, he says, it is now difficult for cardiologists and specialists in dialysis to find jobs.

As medical education moves increasingly toward broader, evidence-based modalities — the science of randomized studies, what's better overall for a group of test subjects — Panisko insists there is still a genuine need for the Herbert Ho Ping Kong art-of-healing approach. "He's dealing with the individual, focussing on the human journey of the patient to highlight memory and teaching points. Tying the emotionality of the anecdote to treatment points improves retention. It can be just as effective."

Dr. MANSOOR HUSAIN

*Dr. Mansoor Husain is the director of the Toronto General
Research Institute, director of the Heart and Stroke Richard
Lewar Centre for Excellence, a senior scientist at the Toronto
General Research Institute and professor of the Department
of Medicine, University of Toronto.*

THE SON OF A PETROLEUM GEOLOGIST, Dr. Mansoor Husain is
both a cardiologist and a scientist. He grew up in Libya, Malta
and Calgary and, precociously, entered the University of Alberta
at the age of 16. After two years of science studies, he was admitted to medical school and graduated as the gold medallist in 1986.
"I did well in medical school and that became a self-reinforcing,
iterative loop," he says. "I continued to do well in part because I
had already done well. I aspired to more and did well, and aspired
to more and did well."

Encouraged to broaden his horizons by leaving Alberta, Husain
won an internship at Stanford University, but turned it down to
do a rotating internship at Toronto's St. Michael's Hospital. He
became chief resident at age 26, then studied cardiology, and did
further post-graduate work in basic science, studying molecular
genetics at Massachusetts Institute of Technology in Boston.

Husain was ultimately drawn to internal medicine for the
same reason many practitioners are — the deep, intellectual challenge it poses. At St. Michael's, he worked under the legendary
internist Dr. Ignatius Fong, a charismatic specialist in infectious
diseases. He says Drs. Ho Ping Kong and Fong, also a Chinese-
Jamaican, represented the British/Canadian tradition of medical
practice, strong on bedside manner. "That was really attractive in
a charming, elegant way. It slowed things down, giving you time

to process the information. But even then, I think, I recognized its limitations."

With the growth of medical imaging, Husain saw, certain kinds of training were no longer as critical. Great clinicians of the past were often able to determine the severity of mitral valve heart disease, for example, by the use of a stethoscope alone. They had a lot of practice, because they would confront, in a career, perhaps 1,000 cases of mitral stenosis. Now, trainees are lucky if they see 50 cases, because there has been a gradual decline of rheumatic heart disease worldwide.

Moreover, medical imaging technology has "completely changed the game of diagnosing the condition." The same technology has changed other specialties as well. "Why would you blindly palpate the abdomen when you can do a CT scan?" Husain asks. His own brother-in-law, a general surgeon, used to appear in the emergency room and automatically lay hands on patients. "Now, he tells me, he just says, 'Have you done the CT yet?' Because there's no way his hand is better than the CT.'"

Husain insists that the laying on of hands — the traditional approach of a doctor to patients — continues to have inherent therapeutic and bonding value. But as a diagnostic tool, it lacks the sensitivity or specificity of scanning technology.

It takes time, typically an hour, to take a new patient history. With older patients, dealing with more complicated conditions, "trainees today may not have the time that is needed," Husain says. "A skilled doctor knows how to take shortcuts and elicit that information, but not the trainee. Indeed, the argument is that there is so much to learn in any one subspecialty than you can't afford the time to spend in general medicine. Therein lies the dilemma. What becomes of the renaissance physician and what will the legacy be? I don't know the answer."

Husain also identifies other troubling consequences of technological change. It's virtually impossible for the mind to absorb the reams of new scientific and medical information that pour forth from scholarly journals and research institutions. Instead, there is Wikipedia. Increasingly, he says, "nobody actually knows anything. They just Google it. That's what's happening and it's happening on the rounds."

Before, doctors needing to confer with a colleague had to physically find them. There were no cell phones. If they needed additional information about a disease or drugs, they had to visit the library and know how to look it up.

"Now," Husain notes, "everything is at your fingertips, like never before. Every piece of information you might need is accessible on your tablet or phone. There's no longer any excuse for not knowing something. But we are short of the time and space needed to bring it all together, to synthesize. You don't need to retain it — why bother? But having access to all the information also means we are expected to deliver instant answers."

The larger question, Husain suggests, is how does one retain the knowledge bank of what is required to be a good physician, without all the memorization of which previous generations had to be capable. "Memory was the reason I did so well in medical school," he concedes. "You can't teach memory, but it is possible that technology has replaced that burden or borne some of it."

Even harder to teach is synthesis — using logic to put ideas together and solve problems. "I don't think technology has yet, and I emphasize *yet*, replaced the human mind in terms of logic and synthesis," he says. "But that's where these software programs are headed. But relying on algorithms to make medical deductions means that there will be no laying on of hands, no actual talking to the patient and getting a sense of how much of his or her complaint is being embellished or whether there is excessive stoicism — not enough disclosure of symptoms."

With the great clinicians Husain has known and worked alongside, including Dr. Ignatius Fong and Dr. Herbert Ho Ping Kong, the tendency is to be overwhelmed by their prodigious feats of memory. But in fact, their greater skill, he insists, is the ability to communicate and connect. "There aren't many idiot savants in medicine, because it's inherently a human skill."

When leading medical students on rounds, Husain makes a practice of role modelling the bedside approach, asking patients about their work and their families. And he takes time after the interview with patients to point out to interns and residents that, even when he has not come up with an extraordinary diagnostic insight, a human connection has been made and that learning has occurred — from doctor to patient and from patient to doctor. "I will leave the room and say, 'You realize why that was important . . . because this patient's job prevents him from doing *A*, *B* and *C*, and if we don't help him address that side of it, it won't matter what prescriptions we write.' That's not in any textbook. That can be taught only through the apprenticeship system of medicine."

But Husain is well aware that he remains, professorially, an anomaly. For most students, he concedes, the patient is simply a symptom or a lab result.

In one of his books, writer and surgeon Atul Gawande — he practises at Brigham and Women's Hospital in Boston and teaches at Harvard — recommends that doctors, no matter how busy or how exhausted they might be, try to connect with every patient on a non-medical level and learn something new about them to prevent fatigue and the effects of the grind.

"That's very insightful," says Husain. "It's really much more for the physician than the patient, but it does help in bonding and establishing trust. The patient sees that 'This man cares for me as a human being.'"

Sometimes, the questions posed may yield medically relevant information — does the patient's lifestyle assist or inhibit his or her ability to follow a diet, rehab or pharmaceutical regimen? But Gawande's point is that even the non-utilitarian question has value, if not for the patient, then for the doctor. "It is refreshing," says Husain. "You get re-energized in your desire to help that individual, just by learning a little more about them."

Ironically, just as the human factor seems to be receding in medical care, patients need it more. They are, after all, confronted by a system that is increasingly dependent on technology, often subject to long, dehumanizing wait times and attended by physicians who are too pressed for time to provide much succour. Moreover, patients — especially the elderly — are battling diseases that are increasingly complex, often requiring them to take a confusing smorgasbord of drugs.

Husain says he makes a practice of telling patients, after his first meeting, what he thinks may be wrong, even before he has sent them for tests, and even if it might be bad news. It is, he suggests, a way to reduce their anxiety, rather than dispatch them to a possible limbo of serial appointments and tests with various specialists. "I think it's important to take them through the possibilities, the differential diagnosis. Here's what I think we may find . . . if it's *A*, we'll do this. If it's *B*, we'll do this. Et cetera.' That's therapeutic, practically. That's important. It shows them that you have connected, that it's not all technology."

When Husain was an intern, telling the patient what you thought was called medical paternalism. In some ways, he now believes, "We have probably swung too far away from that. I'm not sure whether it's driven by fear of legal-medical retribution — being sued — or by the anxiety of just being wrong and recognizing limitations."

But for himself, Husain says he's prepared to say to patients, "'I think I'm 80 percent right' or whatever the percentage it is. It's not based on the latest studies, but simply on a desire to communicate certainty versus uncertainty. That's what makes patients anxious — uncertainty. To quantify it is important. Some people will fret about it and you have to gauge that, with each patient. There's no cookie-cutter approach."

Husain thinks the model of excellence in clinicians will inevitably change. "Maybe the next generational version of Herbert Ho Ping Kong will be someone with all the greatest apps on his iPhone and a great personality, someone who can integrate all the technological advances and knows the advantages and limitations of imaging. A hybrid form, in other words."

Resisting the suggestion that the modern world has made diseases more complex, Husain offers another view: that because our knowledge of biology has expanded, we better comprehend the multi-faceted nature of many diseases. The reality, he says, is that biology lies at the core of many diseases.

"With time, biological systems degenerate," he notes. "We are machines. We wear out. Arthritis, heart failure, dementia — all are degenerative diseases. If you understand the biological principles of degeneration, you will understand all of those diseases. Genetic and environmental influences explain why some people degenerate faster than others. The current excitement about stem cells and regenerative medicine is really an attempt to thwart degeneration. Because if as a child, you break your leg, it will regenerate and you'll never even know it was broken. If you are 90 and you break a leg, you are in big trouble."

Another one of what Husain calls his big concepts focusses on immunology. In medical schools, the subject is seldom taught for more than a month. Most doctors have only an elementary grasp of its principles. Yet, he maintains, it is one of the foundational mechanisms of disease. Autoimmune disorders such as lupus, osteoarthritis, rheumatic fever and polymyalgia rheumatica are essentially immune system diseases.

The body's most important organ, vis-à-vis immunity, is neither the skin nor the lungs — it's the stomach. "It's the first line of defence, because we put things in our mouths," Husain says. Gastroenterology, he predicts, will eventually become immunology because it is microbes, a complex function of what we eat, and our immune system, that determine many of the diseases that affect us. "Vulnerability to coronary heart disease and high blood pressure are dependent on the bugs in you. So it's not just your DNA that matters, but the DNA of every bug in your body, and how it interacts with your DNA."

This, Husain believes, is the medical horizon, and it troubles him. "How do you keep teaching the bedside manner and the human touch when you have to continuously integrate all this new information? People who are conceptually at the leading edge of understanding this nexus of biology and medicine typically don't learn this material until you finish your fellowship — the final polishing-off phase."

Although he studied sciences almost exclusively in school, Husain endorses the notion that a background in the humanities makes for a more well-rounded physician. "I don't feel I missed out big-time, by not reading literature and history. Most stories are derivative, either of the Bible or of the Greek and Roman fables and myths. If you understand those stories, you are connected as a human being. If you are a logical thinker who understands human beings and their vices, then the rest, the science, is pretty easy. It's where some doctors fall down. They have the science, but are lacking the human understanding."

CHAPTER 6

The ART
of PALPATION

Medicine is not only a science; it is also an art. It does not consist of compounding pills and plasters; it deals with the very processes of life, which must be understood before they may be guided.

— Paracelsus

ALTHOUGH IT MIGHT BE CONSIDERED a relatively minor aspect of the clinical examination, the art of palpation — using human touch to assess the patient — is, in fact, one of the most useful skills a physician can develop. It was certainly an important part of the old British system of training. We were well tutored in the art. This included learning how to feel for the shape, size, firmness and loca-tion of key organs and their spatial relationships to other organs.

And not only organs. There is great deal to be learned from any mass that might develop. Is it smooth or rough? Is it hard or soft? Does it move with breathing or is it fixed? Is there lymph node involvement? Does it pulsate? The answers to these ques-tions can tell you a great deal about whether the mass is benign or malignant and, if the latter, how far it has progressed.

In most cases, palpation will be just one of many tools used for diagnosis. But there are times where touch alone can tell you everything you initially need to know. I had occasion to learn this lesson very early in my career. And the patient, as it turned out, was my own father, Percy Ho Ping Kong.

I was in the middle of internship in Jamaica in 1966. My father, only 49 years old and in seemingly good health, complained to me one day about having found dry red blood in his stool. I mentioned this to my good friends, Karl Massiah, a gold medallist in surgery from Barbados who became an orthopedic surgeon, and his wife, Pamela DaCamera, a gold medallist in pathology. Almost in unison, they said my father needed to have a colonoscopy, to rule out bowel cancer. We were fortunate to have Dr. David Atkinson, a fully trained surgeon from Britain working as senior registrar of the hospital. I went to see him.

"David," I said, "my father is experiencing some rectal bleeding. There's no history of colon cancer in the family, but we want to rule it out. He had been diabetic, but he lost weight and is now in generally good health, though he had a sore throat last week."

Atkinson readily consented and in due course arranged for my father to be physically examined. The doctor went through the conventional physical exam and, using his hands, found a lymph node in my father's neck. Later, he performed the colonoscopy, which revealed that my father's bleeding was being caused by inflamed hemorrhoids, more commonly known as piles. Happily, there were no colon polyps and no cancer.

So we were left with the node, discovered in a routine palpation preparatory to the procedure for which my father was being examined, and the week-old sore throat. My two friends were with me to receive Atkinson's report.

"Your dad is from China," they correctly noted. "He could have nasopharyngeal carcinoma." A cancer of the upper throat, the disease is common in South China, with average rates of 25 cases in a population of 100,000 (compared to 1 in 100,000 among North Americans). I would later make this diagnosis on half a dozen of my own patients, all with southern Chinese roots.

It's a disease triggered by the Epstein-Barr virus, the same one that produced lymphoma in Africans.

The next day, my father saw Dr. Wright, a British ear, nose and throat surgeon, who performed a biopsy of the pharynx. It confirmed the diagnosis of nasopharyngeal cancer, a potentially lethal disease. Indeed, in Jamaica, the average patient with this condition lived only six months. Another colleague, neurosurgeon Dr. Andrew Masson, urged me to immediately take my father to London's Royal Marsden Hospital for treatment, and to see Dr. M. Lederman, the world's ranking expert on this particular cancer.

Within 72 hours, my wife, then 32 weeks pregnant, and my father and I were on a plane to London, carrying the various test results. When we met Lederman the next day, he told us my father would have a 25 percent chance of survival. And for every year of survival, his odds would improve by 25 percent. Even though the malignant node had been found on only one side of my father's neck, Lederman believed in radiating both sides. My father spent six weeks in London receiving treatment. As it happened, we knew another Chinese man in Jamaica who developed the same disease; he was radiated on only one side of the neck and died within six months. My father survived his cancer ordeal and lived another 30 years, before succumbing to a heart attack. All of this, remember, was the result of simple palpation procedure performed by a physician who did not automatically assume that because my father was in need a colonoscopy, the lymph node examination was unnecessary.

EXCEPT FOR OBSTETRICIANS AND MIDWIVES, palpation has become a somewhat neglected art. But a good pair of hands can help clinicians reach conclusions and diagnoses much faster and more accurately.

I recall one particularly instructive example. I had been treating a young woman for a condition known as paroxysmal atrial tachycardia (PAT), a particular form of arrhythmia. Not uncommon in young women, and usually caused by some aberration in the heart's electrical conduction system, it yields pulse rates of up to 200 beats per minute. One day, she came to see me with her husband, Howard, a 40-year-old businessman who was on his way to Asia via Los Angeles for a buying trip. In fact, he was planning to leave for the airport in a few hours. He, too, had been my patient.

In passing, he mentioned to me that he had found something suspicious on his private parts, but intended to deal with it when he returned in six weeks.

I said, "This will only take five minutes. Please undress."

I conducted the examination and quickly found a hard lump on his testes.

"You probably won't be going to Los Angeles," I said.

The next day, he saw an urologist who surgically removed the lump. It proved to be malignant. He had lymphoma. We immediately started a course of chemotherapy.

Howard survived for 10 years, before succumbing to a treatment-related lymphoma. This is a common and tragic consequence of radiation and chemotherapy — the malignancy recurs, often in a more lethal form.

Again, I can't stress enough the importance of these simple examination procedures. I can't say whether palpation at an earlier stage would have saved Howard's life, but I do think it's a skill that is too often neglected in routine medical examinations.

SOMETIMES IT IS INTERESTING TO compare notes with patients — to see how they remember the story of their illness versus how I remember it. Quite frequently, it illuminates the truth reflected in the great Japanese film *Rashomon*, by director Akira Kurosawa, which tells the same narrative through characters' different points of view.

Arthur G., whom you will meet below, represents a small version of the *Rashomon* idea. I will let Arthur tell his story first and then provide my own recollections.

A PATIENT'S PERSPECTIVE — *Arthur G.* ——————————

I was raised in a small town in Saskatchewan — population 800 people — halfway between Regina and Saskatoon. My family, the local entrepreneurs, ran the town's hotel and restaurant, the movie theatre, the newspaper. My father died of pancreatitis at the age of 37. I was eight years old. My mother, as he was dying, was coming out of the hospital with my new baby sister.

I worked in the hotel growing up. I was encouraged to go to university, earned a degree in sociology and psychology at the University of Saskatchewan, went to Europe, got a teaching certificate in Alberta, taught elementary school there and then moved to Vancouver. By then I was married, but gay — and eventually I could not avoid coming to terms with that. My wife and I divorced, and I went to back to school to study marketing and corporate communications.

In 1983, I arrived in Toronto just as the AIDS crisis was gathering steam. But I did reasonably well as a producer of sales videos and corporate events. I am today 61. And I met Gilles, my partner, who's in the corporate travel business. We've been together 23 years. We recently sold our house and moved into a condo because of my arthritis. Some days, I can barely walk.

I started drinking when I was 12, stealing liquor from my parents. A nip of this, a nip of that. In high school, bootleggers would buy beer or whatever for us and we'd drink at parties. University was party central and I could party with the best of them. I was not a troubled drunk. I held it very well. Later, when I joined the work force, I'd get home from work, and have a scotch or a few scotches. I just liked the taste. Booze was nice. It would loosen you up. But people would be surprised to know that I had a drinking problem. It wasn't until the last 10 or 12 years that I recognized it. I knew I was drinking too much. My partner occasionally suggested I cut back. A manager at work once summoned me to her office; another colleague had mentioned I smelled of alcohol. I guess I was a functioning alcoholic.

The drink of choice for years was vodka. One drink to start and then free pour and mix. Then some wine with dinner, then smoke a joint. But apart from pot, coffee and alcohol, no other hard drugs. By the time I was diagnosed, I was close to the point where I needed to buy a bottle of vodka every two days.

I developed what I thought was a skin rash and went to see my GP. It looked like red pimples that were spreading. My GP gave me antifungal ointment, but that didn't work, so I went back, because it was getting worse. So he sent me to see a dermatologist, Dr. Barbara Ho Ping Kong, who turned out to be Herbert's wife. This was 2010.

She looked at the spots and said, "Do you know what cirrhosis is?"

I said, "What do red spots have to do with cirrhosis?" Stupid question of the day.

"Do you drink a lot?" she asked me.

"What's a lot?" A standard line I used.

She said, "These are spider veins."

Apparently, the fine ends of your blood vessels are exploding and leave a little scar where the blood has drained. They are an indicator of liver disease. She suggested that I see her husband. So I came here a week or two later to see Herbert and his retinue of interns, humble servants of the wise doctor. And they tap and feel and pluck. I recall no pain, except for my lower back, which is an arthritic condition I have had all my life. Although I was a good swimmer as a youth and worked as a lifeguard, I would throw my back out every once in a while. Now, there are issues with both the cervical and lumbar spine, plus scoliosis, plus degenerative disc disease. On an MRI, my lumbar spine looks like the letter C. I treated it with a lot of opioids. I used to take over-the-counter anti-inflammatories, two or three every morning. I wonder how much damage that did to my liver, long-term.

So by the time I saw HPK, I already had a preliminary diagnosis. One test had showed what they call a grey liver — a sign of damage. My GP had lectured me. I ignored his advice not to drink. I knew that it would turn up eventually, but never thought I'd be exposed by asking about red spots.

HPK confirmed the diagnosis. It was definitive, very firm. I totally got it. But it was delivered in a non-combative way. I did not feel I had been slapped down — "You stupid man. You should know better." He just made it clear that this was the reality. "You have to stop and can't drink, ever again. Or you will kill yourself."

One of his interns said afterward that while that may seem pretty tough, it's easier to quit drinking than quit smoking. And I had already quit smoking. So I quit. I gave myself permission to finish the last bottle of vodka and to take as much time finishing it as I wanted. I finished it that week, and have not had a drink since. Today, my liver has some scarring, which is likely permanent, but my spleen has gone down in size. HPK says he can still feel cirrhosis on the liver, but no fluids, which is good. My blood is fine. If I needed surgery for my back, I'd be okay. My right hip is arthritic and I'm waitlisted for hip replacement. But I'm in pain all the time.

Quitting drinking was not hard. No DTs, no trauma,

no shaking. I got the shakes when I was drinking, every morning when I woke up, when my body was telling me it needed alcohol. HPK wanted me to go to AA, and I said no, it's just not for me. It's about God and God's powers, and I don't believe in that, though I see the value in having someone to run to for help. I knew if I were in trouble, I could call HPK and he'd be on my side. Gilles, my partner, still drinks, but moderately. I used to drink my vodka with lemonade and soda water. Now, at parties, I just have the lemonade and soda water. It lacks a bit of bite.

An interesting thing. The last time I was in Saskatchewan, the fellow who had bought my grandparents' house in town tells me my grandmother left a box behind. He could never bring himself to throw it out. "Would you please come and get it?" So I open it up and what do I find included among the artifacts? This buckle-like thing, etched with the words, "Easy does it. First things first." And the date, 1947. It belonged to my grandfather. The phrases are used by Alcoholics Anonymous. So I brought it home and, while I don't go to AA meetings, I use it as my talisman. Now, it's not just about not drinking. I carry it with me whenever I go out. It's like carrying keys. I told HPK about it and he said, "Whatever works."

Truth be told, I never would have thought that quitting would be so easy. I think part of what kept me drinking is the fear that quitting would be too hard, that I'd be a failure. My view is, "moderation in all things, including moderation." It's useless without the other part, the ability not to be moderate. But you need the wherewithal to control it. Some alcoholics can.

I think HPK saw that this was my way of fighting my addiction and he was very accepting. I was right up his alley, because he believes in listening to the patient. He doesn't talk much philosophy with me, but he's such a gentle soul that you can't help but be straight with him. You don't find people like him that much anymore. He was just so understanding, yet I knew he was totally serious and would not give me the time of day if I came in here with alcohol on my breath, or if he saw something in the blood work. And who could blame him?

ARTHUR HAD BEEN SENT TO me by my wife, Barbara, who had examined him in her dermatology clinic. Her report said he had spider naevi (broken blood vessels) and thrombocytopenia, a low platelet count. These are well-recognized characteristics of cirrhosis patients. A low platelet count can be caused by other conditions such as idiopathic thrombocytopenic purpura (ITP). I had no idea initially that he was a serious drinker. Nor did Barbara, in my recollection. She sent him because of the low platelet count, which was about 60,000, instead of the normal 200,000.

However, when I took his personal history, he readily acknowledged that he was a drinker. And when I performed the physical examination, I quickly established that his liver was enlarged. It felt firm and cirrhotic. He also had an enlarged spleen. All of these indicators taken together — the spidery veins, the low platelets and what I had learned from palpation, the firmness of an enlarged liver and the enlarged spleen — made the diagnosis relatively simple. Ultrasound tests later confirmed it. With practice, you can actually feel the irregular surface of the organ through skin, subcutaneous tissue and muscle. Still, feeling the liver is a sophisticated procedure. One of the finest physicians I ever saw perform this procedure was Toronto Western Hospital's Dr. Ken Robb. He examined a patient that had been feeling unwell, with weight loss and sweating. "The liver has a ground glass feeling to me," he said, after palpating the organ. "This is likely going to be amyloidoisis." And so it proved to be. Amyloid is a very difficult diagnosis to make, but Robb did it merely by palpating the liver.

THE ART OF PALPATION CAN be important in diagnosing any number of conditions. I recall being summoned to the emergency room one night to examine a 70-year-old woman who was feeling generally unwell — not eating and losing weight. The attending ER residents weren't sure what was wrong. Her physical exam looked normal. She appeared mildly anemic, but there was no evidence of enlarged lymph nodes in the neck or elsewhere. The challenge in the emergency room is to develop a reasonable clinical diagnosis and do tests to confirm it. You need to do this well, or else you can waste time pursuing the wrong track, putting the patient at risk. Some medical residents surmised that she might have a neoplastic condition — a tumour somewhere in the body. Others thought it might be tuberculosis.

I then conducted the examination, palpating the liver, stomach, spleen and lymph nodes. There's also a palpation test one can perform for a patient with a thin habitus, or body type, in which you feel the retroperitoneum, the anatomical space in the abdominal cavity, behind the peritoneum. With experience, you can sometimes feel through the skin, fat and subcutaneous tissue for lymph node swelling or Hodgkin's disease. I palpated the area and felt no retroperitoneal lymph nodes, but detected a small, hard nodule at the umbilicus. I turned to my colleagues.

"This person has Sister Marie Joseph's nodule," I said, "and it is evidence of an abdominal carcinoma."

Named for Sister Mary Joseph Dempsey, a surgical assistant of Dr. William Mayo at St. Mary's Hospital in Rochester, Minnesota, in the late 19th century, the nodule protrudes into the umbilicus as a result of metastasis. It is typically a grave diagnosis. The patient I examined likely had an advanced form of ovarian cancer.

So palpation can be a critical tool for diagnosis, although before disclosing it to the patient, you should further test your theory using CT scan and then confirm the diagnosis by biopsy.

One relatively common condition that lends itself to diagnosis by palpation is the abdominal aneurysm, particularly in older patients. You can actually feel its pulsation. The key objective is to accurately measure the dimensions of the aneurysm, which is effectively a bulge in the arterial wall. Three centimetres is considered normal; anything in the vicinity of six centimetres will require surgical repair. Again, ultrasound and, if necessary, the CT scan are invaluable tools for determining the precise dimensions. Palpation can lead you to doing the appropriate tests.

Some 30 years ago, I had a patient with a moderately enlarged goiter, a swelling in the neck usually associated with iodine deficiency. Curiously, she felt no pain at the site of the goiter itself. Instead, the pain was localized in her left arm.

"It is very, very painful," she told me. "It feels like it's beating, doctor."

I put my hand on the arm and could feel the pulsation. It felt deep to me, deeper than the muscle. It was the bone itself that was throbbing.

I feared that its depth suggested cancer, which unfortunately proved to be the case. The formal diagnosis was follicular thyroid cancer, a very vascular cancer that has a propensity to metastasize to bones and the lungs. We tried to reverse its course with radioactive iodine treatments, but unfortunately it was too late.

PALPATION WAS THE ORIGIN OF another diagnosis that did not lend itself to treatment. The patient was Walter, a 42-year-old man who, 25 years earlier, had been successfully given radiation and chemotherapy for Hodgkin's disease. Effectively cured, he was carefully followed for many years. He came to see me complaining about a lump he had found in his lower, anterior chest, just below the breastbone. His family doctor thought it was likely a sebaceous cyst, but wanted another opinion.

The lump was visible — the size of a golf ball — and it was

hard. Just feeling it, I thought it was likely a cancer. As it turned out, it was — a treatment-related sarcoma, induced by the radiation Walter had received a quarter century earlier. It was located precisely at the junction of the protective shield worn during treatment and the rest of his body. Sadly, this is a not uncommon legacy of radiation therapy.

Before making a formal diagnosis, I spoke to a hematology colleague.

"I think I have a patient with treatment-related cancer," I said.

"Where's the tumour?"

"Just below the breastbone."

"That's exactly where they occur," he said. "The area near the edge of the protective mantle also gets radiated."

THE POPULAR PRESS THESE DAYS often carries stories about the coming wave of a diabetes crisis. I wish I could say that these reports are exaggerated, but I suspect they are not. More and more, we are seeing evidence of what physicians call insulin resistance, which is a precursor to full-blown type 2 diabetes, the kind that strikes adults. Such patients have a propensity not only to become diabetic, but to develop lipid disease, coronary heart disease, hypertension and stroke. It's called Syndrome X and it's a major problem. If there is no intervention and change in dietary and exercise habits, a high percentage will develop one or more of these conditions.

One of the clinical features of insulin resistance is a condition known as Acanthosis nigricans (AN), which is characterized by blotches of darkly pigmented skin under the arms, the breasts, in the groin and other folds of the skin. Because of the discolouration, it is not difficult to diagnose. The question is — does the condition suggest that something else might be going on?

I recently saw a 42-year-old Middle Eastern woman with AN. Her endocrinologist had made the initial diagnosis and was concerned about an underlying ailment. That's because the disease is frequently associated with paraneoplastic condition — i.e., a cancer. It's one of those dermatological manifestations of internal malignancies, in the same group as intractable itching.

However, the endocrinologist found no evidence of insulin resistance — the woman had been a competitive skier in her youth and was still fit — and thus sent her to see a gastroenterologist, to look for cancer. When both the gastroscopy and a colonoscopy proved negative, she was sent to see me. I took a full history, as I usually do, and a complete physical exam.

In addition to the Acanthosis nigricans, the skin on the palm of her hands had become coarse and roughened — this is known as tripe palms — and her lips deeply furrowed, known as ruga. Dr. Sanjay Siddha, a dermatological colleague of mine at Toronto Western, later said these were simply other expressions of the same ailment, the most severe he had ever seen.

More ominously, using palpation, I found a series of four or five masses in her abdomen, each as large as a small orange. So her AN was indeed a secondary consequence of an internal malignancy, probably ovarian cancer. The diagnosis of borderline ovarian malignancy was confirmed later by biopsy. The prognosis is uncertain. Some patients can survive for many years, although the skin conditions are intractable.

Obviously, clinicians conducting abdominal examinations of women must be vigilant about protecting the patient's privacy, but it can and should be done. A physician's hands constitute a powerful diagnostic tool. With practice, you can feel and assess the spleen, the liver and the retroperitoneal nodes. In most cases, palpation will be just one of many skills needed to make a proper diagnosis, but I hope these cases demonstrate how pivotal and valuable that art can be.

A

RADIOLOGIST'S

PERSPECTIVE

Dr. ANTHONY HANBIDGE

Dr. Anthony Hanbidge is a diagnostic radiologist at Toronto Western Hospital and an associate professor of medicine at the University of Toronto. He meets with Dr. Ho Ping Kong every Wednesday afternoon to discuss imaging studies from Dr. Ho Ping Kong's internal medicine clinic.

RAISED AND EDUCATED IN IRELAND, Dr. Tony Hanbidge practised family medicine in the small town of Botwood, Newfoundland (population about 3,000), for eight years. "It was fulfilling, but all consuming," he says. "You were never off call. Everyone knew you and where you lived. That's good and bad. You were expected to be always available."

At 30, Hanbidge decided to specialize. He thought seriously about internal medicine. "The idea of disease as a puzzle that had to be solved appealed to me." But he ultimately settled on radiology, because he had developed something of an expertise at Botwood Cottage Hospital. "I was particularly drawn to it. Among my colleagues, I had become the go-to person for reading x-rays."

But when he began talking to admissions personnel for specialization programs, he was effectively told, "You're over the hill. Don't waste our time and your money. You probably won't be successful elsewhere, either."

"That motivated me," he says, "rather than discouraged me."

When he arrived in Toronto in 1990, Hanbidge was stunned to see the degree to which technological innovation had revolutionized his field. "In fairness, I didn't even realize what radiology was. The technological leap was nothing but staggering. Computers were everywhere, and cross-sectional imaging was well established. In 1990, the entire province of Newfoundland might have had two CT scanners, whereas downtown Toronto alone had 10 or 12, perhaps more, plus MRI machines."

For Hanbidge, it constituted a dramatic shift in what he had understood as the practice of medicine. The trend has only accelerated; the use of CT and MRI scans for diagnostic purposes has grown exponentially.

"The technologies are fantastic," Hanbidge acknowledges. As an intern in Dublin, he often assisted at diagnostic laparotomies — exploratory surgery to locate the cause of a patient's pain. "The patient would have had a barium enema, a barium swallow, an intravenous pyelogram and other tests, but in the end, nobody was quite sure what was going on, so we'd say, 'Let's look in there,' and you'd be on the table. You don't see that happening anymore. Technology has delivered the potential for fast and accurate answers."

Today, if a patient presents in a hospital's emergency department with pain in the abdomen or elsewhere, the reflex response is to order an imaging test. In part, that's because of the success of scanning technology in diagnosis. And in part, it's because of the pressures on the emergency department — the overload of patients and the consequent shortage of time. In the past, it was commonplace for surgeons to remove appendixes simply because it was the assumed source of a patient's pain. Today, very few are removed without preliminary imaging studies.

Technology has impacted medical practice in other ways as well. Years ago, if doctors could not diagnose an illness, a patient would often be admitted to hospital and kept under observation. "The thinking was, 'Let's see how he is in six hours or 12 hours or 18 hours,'" says Hanbidge. "You were either getting better, or getting worse or staying the same. Time itself could help provide a diagnosis. Now, using ultrasound, CT or MRI scanners, decisions are made almost immediately, usually before surgeons are consulted. That's a fundamental shift."

But while accurate diagnoses are typically being made much faster, something else, Hanbidge maintains, has been lost — the

entire skill set of chatting, listening, observing, assessing, palpating and percussing. "It doesn't happen in the same way," he says,
"for better or worse. So those skills often don't mature to the
same level." In cases where the diagnosis is clear, this loss is not
critical. "With a hot appendix," he says, "the imaging techniques
will be right most of the time."

But what happens if and when the diagnosis is not so clear?
"Maybe the illness isn't all physical, but a little psychosocial, some
depression perhaps, a family history of something or other. So
there is still a need for having a conversation between doctor and
patient, a chat with a doctor who looks you in the eye and is actually listening. That feels good when you are patient because you
know he cares and he's been caring for a long time — he cares
with interest. If you are in the hands of a very experienced clinician who gives undivided attention, that in itself has amazing
healing power and potential."

The challenge for medicine, going forward, Hanbidge argues,
will be to strike the appropriate balance between the unquestion-
able benefits of technology and the human factor — the still irre-
placeable art of medicine. "There is a danger of weighting it too
much on the technology end. The secret is to manage a balance
to keep enough time in the system to make a human connection.
But if these arts are not taught and learned in the same way by
the next generation, if as a trainee I never have the opportunity
to apply these clinical skills and make up my mind on that basis,
because I know, or I think I already know the answer, then what
will happen in the next 10 or 20 years?"

The importance of maintaining the old medical skill set is
heightened, Hanbidge believes, by the increasing complexity of
modern life. People are deluged by information, not all of which
is reliable or true. On the one hand, the birth of internet culture
means patients are much better informed about their conditions than ever before. In some cases, he concedes, "they know
more about their disease than I do. I'm talking about the rarer

conditions. They will have read everything there is to read online, and will be aware of the risks of this or that and are part of a support group with the same or similar ailments."

On the other hand, there is so much information that patients now often form an opinion of their own diagnosis even before they meet the doctor. "It makes it very hard for them to give me an unbiased presentation of their history. They are not lying. But they have self-diagnosed and are emphasizing symptoms that will lead me in a certain direction."

Even the marvels of technology have become, to some extent, a double-edged weapon. "We see lots of stuff on images that are not relevant to your current complaint or future, potential illnesses — lumps and bumps all over the place. So for all the great work we do in solving problems, we also create a lot of problems. We did not find X, but we found A and B and C. What do you do then?"

It was once the fashion, Hanbidge recalls, for senior business executives and professionals to have whole-body screenings. Everyone, of course, is seeking a clean bill of health. One radiologist found a nodule on his lung and was then faced with the question — do I ignore it and wait a few years and see what happens? Or do I intervene now? "So he wanted an answer immediately and had it biopsied. Complications set in. The lung did not expand. Clots developed in the leg and then a pulmonary embolism. Finally, the nodule was removed and turned out to be benign. He'd probably had it for most of his life. He later wrote an article about the experience in which he confessed that he had once been a big fan of whole-body scans, but was now having second thoughts. Aside from the $500,000 he'd cost the health care system, it had not been much fun."

As the population ages, the medical system will be tested in other ways, Hanbidge predicts. "There are collateral considerations that are difficult to sift through. Resources are finite, and there will have to be more discussions about appropriateness criteria, for certain tests. Say you sprain your ankle. When do you need an x-ray and when don't you? Well, we have guidelines for that. Ideally, that would be expanded to other symptom sets. But it is very hard to reach agreement, even in the same establishment."

It's in this context, Hanbidge suggests, that the pendulum may eventually begin to swing back to the art of medicine, if only because the costs of technology become prohibitive. "We have to manage what we have. And maybe the level of care we give to a 92-year-old should be different than the care we extend to a 32-year-old with dependents."

Hanbidge's own father, a farmer, passed away not long ago at the age of 92. In his entire life, he'd been in hospital two days — at age 44 for a hernia repair. "He died at home in the old farm house without a blood test having been done. He was fundamentally intact until three weeks before he died. A family doctor came a couple of times at the request of the children, and a public health nurse came every day for the last 10 days." But not a single diagnostic test was performed, except perhaps using a stethoscope. "For me, that is completely appropriate," Hanbidge says. "As a culture, we have to be willing to accept that there is a time when dying may not be a bad option, provided it is facilitated with comfort and dignity, and support for the individual and those around him or her. That's a tricky conversation. But maybe that's the real art of medicine, helping people come to terms with death."

RHEUMATOLOGIST'S

PERSPECTIVE

Dr. LORI ALBERT

Dr. Lori Albert is the education/clinical coordinator of the University Health Network's Arthritis Program. She is an associate professor, Faculty of Medicine, University of Toronto. She received her M.D. from the University of Toronto in 1988, completed a residency in internal medicine there in 1991 and a residency in rheumatology in 1993.

WHEN LORI ALBERT WAS A junior staff member in rheumatology at Toronto Western Hospital, she was asked to examine a patient of Dr. Herbert Ho Ping Kong — a young man with an unusual rash. "I think Herbert had already made a diagnosis, but he wanted my opinion," she recalls. "I made a broad differential diagnosis," essentially a way of considering all the various possibilities. "One of them was lupus, but I didn't really think it was lupus, so it wasn't high on my list. Then, HPK came along and said, 'It's lupus.' And I said, 'Well possibly, but I think we need to also consider *X* and *Y*, and do tests *A*, *B* and *C*.' And he said, 'It's lupus.' And of course, he was right, even before the tests were ordered. He just knew, even though it was an atypical case, because it was a man, not a woman. He'd seen it before and there was something he recognized."

Albert already knew Ho Ping Kong, of course, having encountered him at regular sessions of Morning Report, an 8 a.m. medical school gathering where trainees were challenged to figure out a diagnosis of a patient admitted to hospital the previous nights. "The junior resident would parcel out the facts of a case, and HPK would give us cryptic clues that we had to decipher," she recalls. "It was a totally intimidating experience. I remember one case dealt with pulmonary edema, fluid in the lungs, which sometimes makes you cough up blood-tinged sputum. His clue for that might be 'Has anyone been drinking a strawberry milk-shake?' But he was very good about praising you if you made the right deduction, and would lead you through your thought process."

Later, Albert says, HPK was responsible for her decision to go into rheumatology. She had planned a career as a hematology oncologist. "I had done all my electives and rotations in hematology and not done any in rheumatology. And one day I was chatting with Herbert, and he said, 'Have you considered rheumatology?'

And I said, 'Not really.'

'Well, have you done a rotation in rheumatology?'

'No.'

He said, 'Let me go talk to Rob Inman'" — a senior rheumatologist who had been one of Albert's teachers. "So then Rob came to talk to me, persuaded me to do a rotation in rheumatology and the rest is history. But it was Herbert's talking to Inman that set me on that path."

What appealed to her about the discipline, she says, was the chance to develop longitudinal relationships with patients, since many rheumatoid conditions are persistent. "And there's a lot of uncertainty, which translates into diagnostic challenges, recognizing the patterns in things and putting weird stuff together as a disease. I love that, and sometimes I hate it and wish I were doing something like cardiology, which is more cut and dried. But I like hearing patients' stories, assembling the clues and finding what I hope is the answer. The answer isn't always the one they want to hear, but our capacity to treat many diseases has improved in the last 10 years because of medication. And when the diseases have a lot of morbidity, you have to provide psychosocial support, especially for young women who are experiencing side effects of prednisone that may be disfiguring."

Among the hardest aspects of the art of medicine, she says, is the delivery of bad news. "Some people have an innate ability for it. They are just better communicators, better able to delve into dangerous areas. In a personal context — at a cocktail party, for example — I would never ask a leading, personal question. But in the clinic, I will, and I don't mind if they cry, because it means we've got to the crux of the problem."

The facility is also enhanced, she believes, if the doctor has life experience to draw upon — having been a patient or tending to family members or friends who were critically ill. "It gives you a better sense of how you'd want physicians to relate to you," she says. "I think you need to be empathetic, but also know that people can cope if you present things to them in the right way. You have to be upfront, but you also need to lend support."

Albert maintains that, in her field at least, disease is generally less complicated than in the past, because it is usually identified earlier. "Rheumatoid arthritis, for example, has changed dramatically even from when I interned," she says. "It used to be incredibly disabling and now it isn't. People would be admitted to hospital for two weeks of bed rest and that just doesn't happen anymore, thanks largely to new drugs."

What has become more complex, she says, is its context. "People's lives are more complex today. They are under pressure at work or in other aspects of their lives. They may be self-employed, and earn enough money to not qualify for free medications, but not enough to be able to afford the $18,000 it costs for the biologic drugs they need." Increasingly, the art of medicine today involves helping patients deal with issues that surround their lives, not just the disease itself.

Treatment is also complicated by the variety of choices now available. "The treatments are effective," she says, "but they all come with a menu of side effects. Being able to explain to a patient the relative importance of these side effects is tough, all the more so because they will likely have read something about the disease on the internet and have some information, but not enough." It's another example of Alexander Pope's famous dictum, "A little knowledge is a dangerous thing."

On the other hand, patients often don't want too much information — though physicians are obliged to provide it — because they find too much data overwhelming. "We used to be able to say, 'Just take this and you'll get better,' but now we can't. We have to explain everything and it has to be a mutual decision. And the more drugs they have and the more co-morbidities [overlapping diseases], the greater the difficulty of choosing the right treatment. So that's the complicated stuff."

All of this, inevitably, requires time — more time than the disease itself. On some days, Albert says she functions as much like a social worker as a doctor. "I don't mind that, but it's hard to manage the time."

The reality of day-to-day practice in rheumatology, as in other disciplines, demonstrates again that the neat algorithmic medical school formulae offered up to diagnose and treat disease are not sufficient. "We all love algorithms," she says. "They're so clean, neat and tidy. If this, then that. Ostensibly, it means it's harder to make mistakes, and you are more likely to follow the correct trajectory. But people become very dependent on them and don't see outside of them."

In effect, the increase of algorithmic-based diagnosis and treatment implies a correspondent decrease in independent, critical thinking. "It's a real art to get people to think critically." The other corollary of algorithm-dependent thinking, Albert adds, is that it effectively takes the individual out of the equation. By definition, if you are simply following the logic of an algorithm, the actual patient — with all of his or her nuances and idiosyncrasies — becomes secondary. "Yet more and more, the students want that," she says. "It's on your device, your smartphone or your tablet, and it's easy to follow and you don't have to remember as much."

Moving students off that pathway is difficult, she contends, "because they are so driven to do well on exams, in order to get the residency of their choice, and the position they want." Although she thinks the clinical skills courses — on interviewing, conflict resolution, ethics and dealing with difficult patients, for example — are quite good these days, medical students, to her "seem somehow jaded. They don't always see the value of these courses and they have to buy into it to derive the benefit, whereas I, in retrospect, wish I had had the opportunity to learn some of this when I was a trainee."

The so-called hidden curriculum, she says, continues to influence the thinking of young doctors. "They hear all the things about how they should be behave, but when they get to the hospital, they see doctors modelling a quite different form of behaviour. Or they encounter the cynicism of an overworked, under-slept resident. They observe that and think, 'That's what it's really like to be a doctor — not this stuff they teach in lectures.' And what they see in role models, in the end, is probably far more important than what they are taught in the classroom."

CHAPTER 7

ENTERING
the GREY ZONE

Cure sometimes, treat often, comfort always.
— Hippocrates

A FEW YEARS AGO, MY former colleague Dr. David Naylor was invited to lecture to the American Osler Society — named, of course, for Sir William Osler, arguably the greatest physician of the modern age. His address provided a trenchant analysis of the two dominant streams of modern medicine. The first is quantitative, evidence-based practice, which, Naylor noted, "is dependent on applying averages and probabilities to individuals, based on inferences from clinical populations." One might reasonably call this the Science stream.

The second, more patient-centric approach line of attack attempts to use all the skills and tools of medicine to determine the right diagnosis, prevention and treatment for a specific "biological profile" — in effect, the Art stream.

But regardless of which approach one uses, the hard reality,

Naylor observed, is "that we remain at sea when it comes to understanding and preventing or treating many diseases."

Naylor made another salient point as well. Even where there is strong evidence that drug XYZ is likely to combat disease ABC, there is no guarantee that what has worked in a clinical study of 300 patients will actually be effective for one more patient — the one you are treating. "These are the Grey Zones of clinical practice where the balance of harms and benefits is uncertain," Naylor concluded. "We are plagued with exponential uncertainty. The more we learn . . . the greater the number of permutations and combinations that might be contemplated in the care of any individual."

In clinical practice, the Grey Zone divides into two distinct domains. In the first are found ailments that yield symptoms — and symptoms, in turn, cause genuine pain or discomfort — but have no specific label or name. As hard as we may search to identify the precise cause of the complaint, we are often left apologizing to the patient. The best we can do in such situations is to help ameliorate the condition.

In the second domain, which I will examine in the next chapter, are illnesses that have a clear physical basis, but, alas, no effective or remedial treatment. Here, the art of medicine can be sharply tested, because the patient may have to bear the burden of the disease for many years. Technology may help us reach the diagnosis but, in these instances, it is no substitute for the care that such patients need.

Many Grey Zone illnesses fall under the broad, autoimmune umbrella. They are problematic because they often present in non-specific ways. And while we have developed considerable expertise in testing for other diseases, blood markers for several autoimmune disorders have proven elusive. Thus, to diagnose lupus, we often use a set of criteria developed by the American Rheumatology Association; if we find five out of 15 possible characteristics, we conclude the patient has lupus.

However, I have seen lupus patients who do indeed exhibit the classic symptoms of the disease — facial rash, vasculitis, pericarditis, pleuritis and sun sensitivity — and yet their blood sample is negative for anti-nuclear antibodies (ANA), one of the key indications of immune system maladies. And I have seen other patients who show all the requisite clinical and laboratory signs of full-blown systemic lupus erythematosus and, at the same time, all the symptoms and signs of rheumatoid arthritis. We call this Rupus.

My point is to underline the extraordinary complexity that clinicians encounter in the world of autoimmune diseases — yet another reminder that, for all the distance modern medicine has travelled in delineating the processes and mechanism of illness, our journey is nowhere near complete.

AFTER MORE THAN 50 YEARS in medicine, it isn't often that I am presented with an illness that I've never seen or heard of before. But such was the case with Larissa, a married woman and mother in her late 30s. For some time before I met her, she had been experiencing crippling, episodic back pain, often just before sleep. The epicentre of her pain was the 10th thoracic vertebra (T10). It was sometimes accompanied by low-grade fever, as well as by some shortness of breath and dizziness.

Welcome to the Grey Zone, that expansive landscape that physicians must learn to navigate with skill and care. In this chapter, I want to focus on one province of that zone — patients that present with clear, verifiable symptoms of illness, but what illness that is remains a mystery.

Stymied to explain the condition, Larissa's family doctor thought it might be arthritis and sent her to a rheumatologist. Incredibly, he dismissed her complaints as figments of her imagination. She quickly sought a second opinion. This time, a series of x-rays was ordered, which appeared to indicate a large lesion on her left lung and another one at T10. Uncertain whether the lesion was malignant, Larissa was quickly dispatched to Toronto's Mount Sinai Hospital for further tests.

No biopsy was conducted but, on the basis of CT and MRI scans, she was told that she had stage 4 lung cancer that had metastasized to the spine — a devastating diagnosis, needless to say. The doctors were responding to what, on the radiological images, certainly resembled cancer. And her other physical symptoms also suggested that cancer might be at work.

Biopsies of the lung and vertebra were carried out. They revealed inflamed fibrous tissue, taken from the lung lesions. Similar fibrous tissue was extracted from the 10th vertebra, but neither mass was cancerous. That was the good news.

The bad news was that Larissa had a rare condition known as inflammatory pseudotumour. This is essentially a term of convenience, because it describes a wide array of illnesses that affect the lungs and other organs, and carries as many as a dozen names, including such tongue twisters as fibroxanthoma and inflammatory myofibroblastic tumour. It's called tumour-like because it looks and behaves like cancer, but is actually something else. But even today, among her team of doctors, there is no clear consensus on what it is. Hence, the Grey Zone: symptoms, signs and pathology without precise diagnosis.

The presence of high levels of inflammation was confirmed by blood readings. Her erythrocyte sedimentation rate (ESR) was 150, versus a norm for women of her age of less than 20. And her C-reactive protein (CRP) reading was 200, the highest I have ever seen (the norm is about 10).

At that point, she was referred to me. I felt badly for Larissa because she was still quite sick. She was close to respiratory failure, breathing at 30 times per minute (versus a norm of 12 to 16), her nostrils flaring with each breath. And I felt badly for her because, in the first instance, she never should have been told she had cancer.

Again, Larissa's story points to our over-reliance on technology. On the basis of lesions shown on the scans, doctors had seen fit to make this incorrect and life-altering pronouncement. It certainly looked like cancer. The growths showed up in both the lungs and the bones. Therefore it had to be cancer.

Well, no. In fact, it did not have to be cancer. And it wasn't cancer. I've seen this exact situation four times in my career. That is four times too many. Doctors need to be careful to tell their patients the truth, even if the truth is that we don't have the answer. Here, it would have been better to say, "It looks serious but, until we biopsy the tissue, we can't be definitive." And if the patient asked, "Is it cancer?" you would say, "It could be, but we can't be sure. That's why we need to biopsy."

A PATIENT'S TESTIMONY — *Larissa T.* ———————

I noticed immediately that Dr. Ho Ping Kong was different. He actually touched my hand and made physical human contact. No other doctor had done that. I could tell he was a kind soul. He watched and listened. He had a different demeanor. I was quite sick and I found his approach quite reassuring.

I had one very serious episode resulting from the use of prednisone. I was on holiday with my family at Disney World and was unable to sleep, at all. I couldn't continue in that state so we came home, cutting the holiday short, and I was admitted to hospital and sedated for a few days. Ultimately, I was diagnosed as bipolar, which may be accurate, though I think the prednisone was the cause. Because we had to cancel the holiday, my children were upset with me. They weren't talking to me. Dr. Ho Ping Kong gave me a few hundred dollars of his own money and suggested I take my family to the zoo. How many doctors would even think of that, let alone do it?

Today, my lesion has shrunk dramatically and apart from the occasional twinge in my chest, I am pain free. I still take prednisone whenever the inflammation rate creeps up, as well as vitamin D, calcium supplements and milk thistle. I see Dr. Ho Ping Kong every four to six weeks and have blood tests regularly.

THE DIAGNOSIS WAS ONE THING. The central question was how do we treat this condition? Something needed to be done because, even at rest, Larissa had trouble breathing and was close, in my judgment, to respiratory failure.

We thus decided on a therapeutic trial — an "n of 1," as it sometimes called. We use such trials with a single patient for whom a diagnosis has been made, or their disease is known, but for whom no easy or obvious pathway for treatment has been identified. There is nothing scientific about it and such a therapeutic approach should never be confused with randomized, controlled trials.

Of course, some benchmarks are needed to measure the success of whatever therapy is applied. In Larissa's case, there were six — reduced pain, a shrinking of the pseudotumour, lowered counts for ESR and C-reactive protein, a higher hemoglobin count and a general improvement in her sense of well-being.

With those objectives in mind, I started her on a relatively high dosage of prednisone, 60 milligrams per day. Positive results were almost immediate, which was encouraging. But after two weeks on the drug, she developed a swelling on her right arm. Our initial thought was that she developed a deep vein thrombosis. However, an ultrasound of her veins showed no clotting. An MRI revealed nothing specific and, after three weeks, it subsided. We maintained the high dosage of prednisone and added methotrexate, which is widely used to mitigate the negative effects of steroids like prednisone. In the fourth week, a similar swelling occurred on her left side. This time, it lasted only two days. We believed we were on the right track.

After three months, Larissa was almost back to normal, free of pain, her lesions had shrunken and she was able to walk a few kilometres each day.

I HAVE USED SIMILAR THERAPEUTIC trials (n of 1) in other cases as well, with equally good results. One case involved Priscilla, a 60-year-old South Asian woman who complained of feeling generally unwell for about six months, with a slight fever and sweating. My initial hypothesis was that it might be a recurrence of an old case of tuberculosis. I took a full history, did a physical exam and ordered tests — chest x-ray, blood work, etc. Everything came back normal. I arranged for a bone marrow test, in order to rule out cancer and to culture for the TB bacillus. But that, too, proved negative. Despite these readings, I still felt that tuberculosis was somehow implicated. If it were TB, several variations were possible — lung TB, bone TB or TB meningitis.

The most likely form, I thought, would be what is known as cryptic miliary tuberculosis, a special form of disseminated tuberculosis. It is termed "cryptic" because it lies hidden and is therefore very difficult to diagnose. In one study, the proper diagnosis was made during life in only seven of 15 cases (47 percent). The name itself derives from the wide distribution of small lesions in the lung that actually resemble millet seed (hence "miliary"). Although the cryptic form is rare, it does tend to strike older women from India and other parts of Southeast Asia.

The more overt form of the disease, miliary TB, is not difficult to diagnose; the classic symptoms include weight loss, profuse sweating, fever and cough. The lesions are typically visible on x-rays and have the appearance of a snowstorm. But some patients do not present in this manner — only with what physicians call a "failure to thrive."

For Priscilla's therapeutic trial, I again established criteria of improvement — general well-being, weight gain, absence of fever, higher hemoglobin counts and a lower ESR (erythrocyte sedimentation rate). We quickly put her on TB medication — standard care includes isoniazid, rifampin and ethambutol — but her stomach did not adapt well to the regimen. Perhaps something else was going on. We then did a test for the presence of H. pylori, the bacteria known to cause stomach ulcers; it came back positive. After we successfully treated Priscilla for that condition, the TB responded well to drugs; within three months, she was back to her normal self.

IN GENERAL, IT IS NOT difficult to enlist the support of patients and their families to participate in such therapeutic trials. After all, they are clearly suffering. Any relief would be welcome and beneficial. At the same time, they understand that it is a trial and that there are no guarantees of success. For physicians, it is critically important to remember Hippocrates' injunction — do no harm. Unless you can establish firm criteria that measure improvement, it will be wiser not to embark on the n of 1 course.

PERHAPS I HAVE A PERSONAL soft spot for Grey Zone diseases because I had one myself. In the early 1990s, I was suddenly hit with feelings of overwhelming fatigue. A variety of tests assured me that I had no formal, identifiable disease, but the condition persisted. I don't know what precipitated it, but it might have been a Caribbean holiday, when I developed diarrhea. Returning to Toronto, I was sick for several days and recall not being able to eat.

For the next six or seven years, perhaps more, I was lethargic and dragged myself around. At the office, I would often seize an opportunity to take short naps in my office. I frequently had a bad taste in my mouth. I just didn't feel right and had to rest for an hour before visiting relatives. This was classic chronic fatigue syndrome, a condition many regard as fictitious or psychosomatic. I do not.

Eventually, I recovered. The symptoms gradually disappeared and I regained my normal levels of energy and activity. My experience underscored for me the importance of what I think is often the best medicine. I call it the tincture of time.

NOT LONG AGO, DONNA, A perfectly healthy 66-year-old retired school teacher came to see me, referred by her family doctor. She had been feeling generally unwell and complained of dizziness and anxiety. On several occasions, she had experienced a rapid heartbeat (tachycardia), and twice had felt compelled to visit a hospital emergency ward. Her blood pressure on those occasions was elevated — 190/120 — and she was sweating. They told her she had experienced a panic attack.

When I saw Donna, she told me that she had not adjusted well to retirement, although she did occasionally travel to the Caribbean island of Grenada to work as a school volunteer with the hearing impaired. I ran a series of tests to check for serious illness and hormonal imbalances. A few rare diseases — including pheochromocytoma, a tumour of the adrenal glands, and carcinoid syndrome, a slow growing tumour of the small bowel — can manifest with panic attacks and over-stimulation of the body's sympathetic nervous system. All the tests, urinalysis and CT scan were normal. However, I did prescribe medications to control her blood pressure and to slow down her heartbeat, which would prevent her from having to visit the emergency room.

After a few visits, I told her that she was fundamentally healthy and that her anxiety would eventually dissipate. All that was needed was the tincture of time. I encouraged Donna to make another visit to Grenada, where she might feel she was making more of a contribution, but that otherwise she should learn to enjoy her retirement, a reward for her many years of service. A month later, she returned. The blood pressure was under control and there had been no further visits to the emergency department. Then she did go off to Grenada and when she returned, six weeks later, she felt cured. And she was cured.

So what was it, in the end? I don't really have an answer. If I had to make a diagnosis, it would likely be labile hypertension (sometimes called serotonin hypertension) that, from time to time, had generated her feelings of panic, sweating and accelerated heart rate. But it was one of those diagnoses that could neither be categorically proven nor disproven.

What I do know is that Donna trusted me — trusted my knowledge and instincts — and I think that was critically important. Beyond that, I would simply say that, every now and then, life presents us with challenges to which the body and the mind react in unpredictable ways. But physicians can, in fact, be helpful and supportive while the patient traverses the tincture of time route.

THESE MOMENTS OF CRISIS CAN happen to anyone. I recall Cynthia, a 35-year-old mother, a former magazine editor with two well-adjusted school-age children and a good marriage. One day she was completely functional and, virtually the next day, she was fatigued to the point of exhaustion. Unable to manage simple chores like shopping, laundry and cooking, she had to take a leave of absence and hire household help.

She had been fatigued and generally feeling unwell for about five years when I saw her. The origin of these ailments is not clear. Often, it seems to be the legacy of a viral illness, but there can be other triggers as well, including bacterial infections or even the trauma of a stressful event, such as a car accident. I had seen that before.

In these situations, I undertake at least a limited workup, to insure that there is no organic condition that might have been missed. It is unwise, I think, to suggest automatically that this must be chronic fatigue syndrome, because the odds are too good that something else may be going on. And I tell patients like Cynthia that while I will do the best I can, there's a good chance we may not be able to make a precise diagnosis. Most accept that caveat, but others occasionally leave with some anger and resentment that we haven't definitively identified the problem.

On examination, the only physical sign of something amiss with Cynthia were cholesterol deposits in the eyes. My instinct was that these were not significant. Otherwise, her tests were completely normal — hemoglobin, iron levels. When it came time for me to render a verdict, I told her that my best guess was that she had contracted a virus of some kind, although it might even have been caused by a stressful event, like a minor car accident.

I also gave my familiar tincture of time sermon. Having been assured that there was nothing seriously physically wrong, she should take comfort in knowing that the virus, if that is what it was, would eventually burn itself out and that she would return to her normal self. I always recommend the adoption of an exercise regimen. It does not have to be punishing, just something regular, regardless of how reluctant you may be or how unwell you may feel. My exercises of choice are walking, swimming, yoga, dancing, tai chi and transcendental meditation.

What I did not do, and what I try very hard to avoid doing, was prescribe anti-anxiety drugs. I will prescribe supplements if I find iron deficiency, but I never recommend anti-depressants. In fact, I discourage their use. If you can recover naturally, why take medication? With drugs like valium (tranquilizers), there are problems with long-term usage, including seizures and a propensity to break one's hips when older. Dementia is also more common in those who become habituated to anti-depressants. If a patient insists on a prescription, I will suggest that they ask a psychiatrist to write it.

I saw Cynthia several times over the course of a year. Like Donna, she went away for a holiday in the sun and when she came back, the dark clouds had lifted. She was better.

However, my aversion to the prescription of anti-depressants should not be construed as a critique of psychiatric treatment. The work of psychiatrists can go hand-in-hand with the work of general internists, especially once it has been determined that the patient is not suffering from any physical illness. Even patients *with* some physical illnesses — cancer and Parkinson's disease, for example — may sink into deep depressions, for which psychotherapy can provide enormous benefit. In fact, at one point, the University of Western Ontario's medical school ran a joint program for the two disciplines, so closely did they perceive the linkages to be.

Nor am I skeptical about the potential efficacy of anti-depressants, when other avenues (exercise, diet, meditation, psychotherapy) have proved of no avail. In cases of severe depression, there is no doubt that chemical treatments do help. For some patients, so did electro-convulsive therapy (ECT), when it was widely used four and five decades ago, though I acknowledge its dangers and risks. Some members of the modern pharmacopeia, such as Prozac, also have incurred bad names in recent years. Again, however, in tens of thousands of instances, it and comparable drugs have been effective in lifting the clouds of depressions so dark as to be immobilizing — and often within a much-compressed time frame.

CHRONIC FATIGUE AND SIMILAR SYNDROMES predominantly affect women, but I have treated men for the same condition.

One, Darren, was a 55-year-old physician who, like Donna and Cynthia, had not been feeling right for several months. He reported palpitations, fluctuations in blood pressure, a general feeling of malaise and problems sleeping. He had a coronary workup, everything short of an angiogram, but nothing suggestive of cardio-vascular disease was found.

When I saw him, he told me he was happy at work and had a good relationship with his wife and children. I conducted a number of new tests, including urine collections for possible evidence of carcinoid and adrenal tumour but, apart from a slightly elevated blood pressure, Darren was fundamentally healthy. I told him he had minimal hypertension, which was not uncommon, and was usually treated with beta blockers.

"How do you feel when you go on holiday?" I asked him.

"I don't know," he said. "But I'm going to Cuba in a few weeks and we'll see."

When he returned, he told me he had been fine in Cuba but the anxiety, palpitations and other symptoms had reappeared once he was home. So I prescribed a beta blocker to slow his heart beat and gently lower his blood pressure and, within a few months, he reported feeling better.

Again, my hunch is that part of their recovery relates to their confidence in me — the belief that I am covering all the bases. The patient is assured that if there is a physical problem somewhere, I will find it. And, just as important, if I do not find it, it means that whatever is causing their anxiety and its indicia will not be fatal, and that it will, in time, pass.

In these situations, I often find myself saying, "You will get better."

The frequent response is "How do you know that?"

To which I say, "I just do."

And occasionally, I will also tell them the story of my own encounter with chronic fatigue.

GREY ZONE CASES ALWAYS POSE a challenge, but particularly to family practice. Most general practitioners are very busy and the time they can devote to any one patient is necessarily limited. Yet with patients who have genuine symptoms, but no easily identifiable malady, it's precisely time that is often needed most — time to talk and listen and win their trust and reassure them.

Not long ago, Sarah G., a former social worker and now a writer, editor and publisher, came to see me with classic Grey Zone symptoms — dizzy spells, fatigue, migraine headaches, unable to do routine stuff, unable to concentrate. Almost inevitably, some mild depression set in. High achievers are not accustomed to becoming so severely and so suddenly incapacitated. An MRI proved normal, as did the other routine exams and blood work. Of course, I took a full family and personal medical history and examined prior medical records. Eventually, I concluded that no organic illness was present, that nothing was being missed. The task, then, was to persuade Sarah that, despite her symptoms, she was essentially healthy and would recover. She needed to eat well, exercise regularly and enjoy her stable family life. Within a few visits, she felt better.

A PATIENT'S TESTIMONY — *Sarah G.* ————————————————

For no apparent reason, I was suddenly sick. It was like flu, but I just did not get better. I was weak and sweaty and weepy. I was very hot, but did not register a fever. I was emotional and not myself. This lasted for weeks.

I was otherwise healthy. My blood pressure is textbook. I eat well. I don't exercise enough, but I don't drink or use drugs. Nothing psychological happened at the time. I just collapsed.

I went the usual route — first to my GP, an excellent doctor who did all the usual tests and more. But I had to keep coming back because I had no life. Eventually, he referred me to a brilliant woman at Women's College Hospital, and she found nothing. She looked for Lyme disease, autoimmune disorders. You are grateful you don't have a horrible disease, but I was still sick, and completely useless. I could pass as normal, but I wasn't. I could still go out and see friends. But I wasn't myself. I cancelled a lot of appointments because I had to be in bed. A year went by and I started to feel desperate. The doctor said I could come back but that she had nothing to add. At least she did not treat me like a mental case, which often happens to women with these complaints.

I knew someone who was working as a consultant with Toronto Western and asked him to ask if there was a Dr. House working there. "I need a genius," I said. "Not just smart." I was having a bad time. I was in bed and depressed and that is not typical for me.

That was how I arrived at Dr. Ho Ping Kong. The first time I saw him, he spent 90 minutes with me. Who does that? I was blown away. I watched him with my professional social worker eyes and it was an extraordinary experience. We chewed the fat. He just got me as a person. He said right then, "You're going to be fine." I continued to see him every three or four months while we did more tests, but he'd always say you're going to be fine. Once, he did so in the presence of a young resident he was teaching. And when HPK said, "You'll be fine," the resident timidly challenged him and asked, "How do you know that she'll be fine? What is the evidence?"

And HPK wasn't patronizing. He turned to him and said simply, "There are still a lot of things about the human mind and body that we don't understand." It was like a variation on Hamlet's speech, "There are more things in heaven and earth, Horatio, than are dreamt of in your philosophy."

There was never any flavour, any sense that that he was

hinting that "it's all in your head." He just repeatedly said I'd get better in time. And I am better. Certainly the trend is up. Until recently I'd have said I was functioning at 95 percent. But I recently spent a week in bed, utterly exhausted, slightly feverish, slightly nauseous, slightly dizzy.

I don't like the word genius but I think HPK is one, indubitably. He has knowledge no one else I have encountered has. It's East and West. It is art and science. I don't have the right words for it, but he has the capacity to look at me and see disease and disorder and weigh it up and yet say you will be okay.

I was a therapist for many years and I know there are therapeutic effects to extending hope to patients. He would say, "I can't tell you why I know you will be better, but you will." And it changed the whole dynamic. So when I have these periods now, I know they will end and they are endurable because of that knowledge. I'm not in pain. I'm not missing work. No one is going hungry. I have one weird thing that makes me slightly less productive. I'm used to writing every day, but I haven't been. It's made me question my commitment to productivity. Who am I working for? So I have this little thing, but in the big scheme of things it's not so bad. I can't complain about my life. It could be a lot worse.

A

PERSPECTIVE

Dr. MOIRA KAPRAL

Dr. Moira Kapral is a senior scientist at Toronto's University
Health Network and an associate professor of medicine at
the University of Toronto. Her research interests include
cerebrovascular diseases, health services research and women's
health. A staff physician in the UHN's Division of General
Internal Medicine and Clinical Epidemiology, she also runs
an osteoporosis clinic and is a scientist with the Institute for
Clinical Evaluative Sciences (ICES).

UNTIL SHE MET DR. HERBERT HO PING KONG, in her fourth year
of medical school, Dr. Moira Kapral had planned a career as a
general practitioner. She became interested in medicine in high
school, drawn by a combination of the appeal of altruism and science. Her original vision was to open an office in an under-serviced
area of Ontario. Ho Ping Kong was then director of the University
of Toronto's internal medicine program, in charge of selecting
students admitted to the post-graduate residencies. "He also led
Morning Report," a form of highly interactive teaching, she recalls.
"We were in awe of him. He made me really excited about internal
medicine, his enthusiasm and his way of practising. So I became
interested in pursuing that field."

Kapral then did a four-year residency in internal medicine
and was named chief resident in her final year. She later completed a master's degree in epidemiology, also at the University
of Toronto.

During her chief residency, she worked closely with Ho Ping
Kong, attending to both in-hospital patients as well as patients
who were part of his private practice. Typically, she says, a patient

would come to see him after having seen several doctors who were unable to make the diagnosis.

"These patients were essentially languishing in the system," she says. "And he would use his art of medicine to figure out what was wrong, usually by thinking of something that had not been considered before, and do a test to confirm it. It was often a test others might not have wanted to pursue, but he did. And it would lead to a diagnosis and a therapy. That happened dozens of times and the patients were so grateful for finally having an answer." Ho Ping Kong's particular gift, Kapral feels, is the physical examination. "He could use that to find things and not have to rely on other technology."

Beyond his medical skill set, what impressed Kapral about Ho Ping Kong was that, with at least 100 trainee residents under his effective command at any one time, he knew them all on a first-name basis and could engage any one of them on a personal level, asking about spouses or partners or children.

But the art of medicine as modelled by HPK, she says, is at risk, threatened by "an increasing reliance on technology and an over-reliance on formulaic medicine and guidelines." In internal medicine, trainees must demonstrate proficiency in clinical medicine and physical diagnosis. That, she says, is at least partly the result of Ho Ping's Kong's leadership of the Canadian Royal College of Physicians and Surgeons committee on Internal Medicine. The standard tends to be less rigorous in other countries.

Technology, Kapral says, constitutes a mixed blessing for modern medicine. On the one hand, it provides ready access to reams of information that may not be in the knowledge base of the attending doctors. "Nobody has a perfect memory," she says, "and, in the earlier era, if you came up against something you weren't sure about, or hadn't read about, you likely would not have had a quick way of finding out about it, and the patient might have suffered. Now, someone can have access to the most up-to-date information and the latest management plan. On a certain level, care is improved by having that ready technological access to excellent information.

On the other hand, she notes, "Sometimes you may not have access or may go to the wrong source or may not have time to research because things are moving too quickly. If you don't have a certain amount of knowledge, you may not be able to treat people properly in the moment."

Kapral says medical schools across Canada are doing a much better job than they once did of teaching the importance of communication and patient involvement in decision-making, as well as the clinical diagnostic skills needed to practise the art of medicine. "The residents I see coming through the system have been well trained in management and advocacy. They are by and large committed and caring."

The challenge for medical students to learn the art of medicine has been made more difficult, owing to changes in the training program. In the past, trainees learned it on the wards, seeing patients, having mentors. Today, she says, there is more didactic learning — lectures or research, so the amount of time they are exposed to patients and to role models like Herbert Ho Ping Kong has been reduced. "Fifteen years ago, a resident would feel responsible for the ongoing care of a patient during their stay in hospital, although there was supervision by a staff physician," says Kapral. "Now, spending several half days off the wards, there is less continuity."

Other changes, such as limits on the number of consecutive hours that trainees can work, also have had an impact. On the positive side, the new rules means patients are less likely to encounter a tired, overworked physician. But they also mean a patient's file is more likely to be handed off to doctors less familiar with their case.

The internal medicine specialists that will ultimately succeed the Ho Ping Kong generation have been, she believes, well trained. And they have been strengthened by developments in technology and the rise of evidence-based medicine. Unfortunately, the relatively ease of access to MRIs and CT scans — and the increasing fear of lawsuits — means that sending a patient for an imaging scan has become almost a reflex. Although the per-test cost of such procedures has declined, "the system probably spends more money than it needs to because of the sheer volume."

In any event, she says, such tests will never replace the art of clinical medicine practised at the bedside or the examination room. "You can't know which test to order until you've done a thorough history and physical exam."

Dr. MATTHEW STANBROOK

Dr. Matthew Stanbrook is an assistant professor in the
Department of Medicine and the Institute of Health Policy,
Management and Evaluation at the University of Toronto;
associate editor of the Canadian Medical Association Journal
(CMAJ) *and a staff respirologist at the Asthma and Airway*
Centre of the University Health Network.

BORN AND RAISED IN TORONTO, Matthew Stanbrook was always fairly confident he would end up in medicine — in part, he suggests, because his mother was a nurse. But as "the kind of person who always kept my options open," he deliberately spent his first university year studying business, before deciding that the commercial world was not for him. He also briefly considered law, his father's profession. Medicine eventually triumphed and, in preparation, he completed his undergraduate degree at the University of Toronto in pharmacology.

Staying in Toronto for medical school, he expressed an initial interest in trauma surgery. "It seemed glamorous," he explains. But the attraction faded when he was exposed to its harsh realities. "A lot of surgery is tedious and meticulous and careful and that wasn't for me," he says. "I like the process of solving mysteries."

Thus did he end doing his residency in internal medicine, where he specialized in respirology. Apart from the field's many research challenges, Stanbrook had a personal interest — a case of asthma that had plagued him since childhood. The ailment took him to hospital emergency wards on several occasions and, once, he had to be hospitalized for a week.

He found his lectures in evidence-based medicine so fascinating that he decided to pursue a Ph.D. in clinical epidemiology, inspired by public safety physician Ed Etchells and mentored by epidemiological scientist Donald Redelmeier, both at Sunnybrook Hospital. It was Redelmeier who, observing Stanbrook's facility in editing research manuscripts, suggested he get involved in journal editing.

As a result, Stanbrook interrupted his Ph.D. work to spend a year in Boston at the *New England Journal of Medicine* as its first editorial fellow. Today, Stanbrook devotes half his professional life to his work as deputy editor of the *Canadian Medical Association Journal*, a position he's held for six years. "It keeps me current on the breadth of medicine," he says, "and gives me a broader perspective on research."

Despite the critical role played by science in medicine, Stanbrook is also a strong advocate of the art of medicine. "Science is what we largely talk about and study and teach and champion," he concedes, "but it's actually only a small part of what we do. The art is everything else that is not science. Some of that art is taught, some is learned by mentorship and experience, some is innate ability. It's usually a combination. But it's more important than science in what we do for patients. It's most of what we do as physicians. If you don't pay attention to it, you will not be a good doctor. And you will know that — and your patients will know it."

Overwhelmingly, he says, medical trainees that fail or are asked to repeat rotations are not faulted for their lack of knowledge. "It's never on the science. It's on the art — failing to be sensitive to the needs of the patient, not listening, not being empathic." Stanbrook says he learned lessons about empathy and breaking bad news to patients in first-year medicine that "are still with me. And I think the earlier you learn them, the more comfortable you will be in the rest of your clinical training."

How does a doctor optimally break bad news? With a sense of hope, Stanbrook insists. "You may think, 'Okay, I have to tell a patient he has terminal cancer. There can't be anything I can make a difference with.' Yes, there is. What makes the difference is how that news is received and how it is explained and the opportunity you give them to respond and to ask questions."

The way to begin such conversations, he says, is not "with the conventional, 'Hi, how are you today? How's the family?' but much more directly. 'Mr. Jones, we have your test results and they indicate you have a lung cancer.' That's what people need to know. There should be no beating about the bush. Address the issue that's on their mind."

When he is delivering such news, Stanbrook then stops. He doesn't hold forth at length on the details. "I want to give the patient time to respond, to let them set the agenda of questions. 'How far has the cancer progressed? What are the treatment options? How long will I live?'"

To the last, challenging question, Stanbrook suggests it's best to be imprecise. "It's okay to give boundaries. But it's foolish to talk about averages, because it's usually variable and it takes away people's hope."

Communicating bad news, he allows, is the most difficult part of his work. It is especially so when patients are younger. "I had a young man in his 30s, dying of metastatic lung cancer, and he'd done nothing wrong. He'd never smoked. It was just one of these things. So we went from 'There's something wrong, let's do some tests and find out what's going on,' to 'It's metastatic cancer,' and then watched him die within a month. That was one of hardest things I've ever had to do."

Everybody has cancerous cells in them, Stanbrook notes, but the body's active surveillance system finds the deviants and eliminates them. In some people, however, the detection system is faulty or goes awry, usually due to genetic variation or environmental exposure. "There's no justice to it," he says. "It's just life and part of my job, and the part you have to be comfortable with, to go into medicine."

Stanbrook views the profound effects of technology on medicine as a double-edged sword. On the one hand, it has conferred enormous benefits of speed and efficiency, access and dissemination of knowledge and simple communication.

Evidence-based medicine itself, the modern paradigm, couldn't exist without technology, he argues. "I don't mean we haven't had science-guided medicine. I'm talking about a culture shift in which we use the research to inform every decision we make. And that's only possible because we now have efficient ways of sifting. All of medical literature is at our fingertips." The development of those archival tools was, he contends, the necessary precursor to the emergence of evidence-based training as the core conceit of medical schools.

In turn, it created a genuine power shift within the medical establishment. Where medicine had previously been shaped by powerful opinion leaders and sometimes-dogmatic voices of experience, now any first-year medical student could challenge conventional wisdom with empiric justification and guide their own learning. "Those experts are still there," Stanbrook notes, "but they have had to adapt. And it's a crisis for them in a way, because science has had to adapt to this environment. It's raised standards, because science has had to take these extra steps to prove efficacy. It's made research more expensive and difficult, but it needed to be that way."

Proving the law of unintended consequences, the great technological leaps of recent decades have also yielded such an explosion of information, that it has become "increasingly hard to keep up" on current thinking in medicine, he adds. The pressure is even more intense because the same technology has given patients unprecedented access to medical knowledge, enabling them to pose more complicated questions to their physicians.

Some three decades ago, one study showed that, in order to keep abreast of new developments in the field, a general internist would have to spend more time reading than there are hours in the day. The situation is much worse now, Stanbrook says, so you have to instruct trainees not to read journals generally, but to read around their specific patients and use those examples to learn.

"We have to manage a great deal more than we used to," Stanbrook says. "And we have to be managers of information more than ever before." The pace of change is so rapid that doctors are constantly playing a game of catch up. "No one yet fully understands the effect of social media. It may be providing opportunities we are missing or causing problems we aren't even aware of."

It was the exponential growth of medical information, Stanbrook suggests, that created the need for subspecialization. "Gone are the days when a primary care physician can keep up on everything he or she needs to," he says. Does that lead to fragmented care for patients? "It frequently does," he says, "as well as miscommunication and duplication of effort. But if you develop heart disease, a family doctor can do the basics, but it rapidly becomes complicated, and you need a specialist. And having a specialist, study after study shows, makes a difference to patient outcomes."

CHAPTER 8

FURTHER EXCURSIONS in the GREY ZONE

The physician should not treat the disease,
but the patient who is suffering from it.
— Maimonides

IN THE LAST CHAPTER, I REVIEWED a series of cases dealing with the complex challenges that physicians face in dealing with syndromes that cannot be clearly identified, despite the obvious physical and mental suffering they inflict on patients. In this chapter, I will look at a few cases in which we can make a firm diagnosis of physical illness, but offer no effective or lasting solution. Here, the art of medicine is likely to be measured by other factors — by the level of care, attention, empathy and advocacy a doctor brings to the bedside. Sadly, in such situations, it is often necessary to deliver bad news to these patients. But that, too, is an art that needs to be developed.

A FEW YEARS AGO, A COLLEAGUE at a nearby hospital referred a very difficult case to me. Marnie was a 40-year-old woman that had been diagnosed with Erdheim-Chester disease. First identified by two pathologists in the 1930s — Austrian Jakob Erdheim and American William Chester — the syndrome is characterized by excessive production of histiocytes, a type of white blood cell that the body normally deploys to fight infection. When histiocytes over-produce, however, they invade the body's connective tissue and begin to play havoc with key organs, including the heart, bone, kidneys and liver.

The disease is extremely rare: at any time, there are only a handful of cases in all of Canada, and relatively few are described in the annals of medical literature. In fact, when I first read Marnie's file, I had never heard of it. There is no known cause, nor, alas, a cure. Pending a research breakthrough, the best an attending physician can do is to use various drugs to ameliorate the symptoms. These typically include bone pain in the legs and arms, weight loss, difficulty walking, rapid eye movements and bulging eyes, fever, night sweats, muscle and joint aches, weakness and fatigue, excessive thirst and urination.

Marnie's condition generally fit the stereotype. In addition, several years earlier, she had had a pacemaker attached to her heart, the result of what she said had been some 200 fainting spells — actually, they were cardiac syncopal attacks. Although she had been for regular checkups, it seems that doctors had only tested the reliability of the pacemaker itself, not the functioning of her heart. If they had, they would have heard, as I immediately did, what we call a pericardial rub, a murmur that signals inflammation in tissue surrounding the heart. I had no doubt there was a connection between the malfunctioning heart and the bone pain and other problems she was experiencing. Erdheim-Chester was interfering with the conduction system of her heart.

A very intelligent young woman, Marnie became pro-active in using the internet to research her disease and reach out to other sufferers. We tried a number of drugs to ease the symptoms, including prednisone and Enbrel, but nothing seemed to work. In fact, Enbrel caused new and quite acute chest pain, a not uncommon side effect.

Then we learned about a French study that had used Kineret, a drug deployed to treat rheumatoid arthritis, on patients with Erdheim-Chester disease. Two patients had reported positive results. Unfortunately, Marnie's insurance company was initially reluctant to underwrite the costs of Kineret.

The situation speaks to what I think are two other important, but often ignored, aspects of the art of medicine — advocacy and empathy. Obviously, it would be impossible for physicians to spend long hours dealing with insurance companies or other agencies that can and do impact a patient's well-being. On the other hand, you should always want to do the very best you can for the patient, no matter how challenging the circumstances. In that context, knowing how and when to advocate for patients ought to be no less important a part of medical training than knowledge and team-playing.

The same goes for empathy. One can't help being moved by the sight of men and women in the prime of life debilitated by the effects of devastating illnesses. You can't ever afford to let your emotions cloud your judgment, but you will be a better practitioner if you genuinely care and if the patient actually senses that you care. I don't readily cry in the face of the human tragedies that I encounter every day. But I certainly feel their pain, anxiety and confusion deeply inside. And I'd like to think that my patients are aware of my empathy.

In the end, we were able to persuade Marnie's insurers to pay for a three-month trial of Kineret. They agreed to defer a decision on future funding depending on the outcome. Initially, the results were positive, far beyond my expectations. Her pain decreased dramatically. Within two days, this once-bedridden woman felt well enough to shovel snow, although she probably ought to have resisted the temptation. The pain in her chest and legs went from a nine or 10 on a scale of 10 to a far more manageable three or less. For about six months, she was truly her old self. Unfortunately, the effects were finite. Slowly, the drug began to lose efficacy and the pain returned. We then tried another drug, Actemra, which is administered once a month by infusion. At the time, one patient in the United States had experienced some relief with this medication. But the insurers want evidence of efficacy, preferably in trials involving thousands of patients. They agreed to fund it if, after three months, it seemed to be working. So our own Centre for Excellence in Education and Practice paid for the first three months. Unfortunately, it was unsuccessful. We then tried radiation, but that, too, proved unavailing. Sadly, the progress of Erdheim-Chester is inexorable and all that remains for attending physicians is to make the patient as comfortable and pain free as possible.

A PATIENT'S TESTIMONY — *Marnie K.* ————————————————

I was a professional photographer doing family portraiture and landscape, but I had to stop. The disease usually manifests itself as bone lesions, then spreads to the organs and eventually shuts them down. I happen to have the cardiac involvement. It hasn't been classified as a cancer, but it acts like a cancer in the way that it spreads. As far as we know, there is no genetic component. The cause could be environmental. It could be stress. I have had a stressful life.

The pain can be quite intense at times. On a scale of 10, it is sometimes a 15. And I've given birth, so I know what pain is. There is no medication proven to be effective. There are pain management techniques, but I am allergic to the whole family of opiate drugs. Morphine, Vicodin, Percocet are all off limits for me. It became very difficult to continue working.

It started in my legs. I began an exercise program and noticed pain. I went to see my family doctor, who ordered x-rays and they did show a single-unit mass extending far up my leg. Then I went to see an orthopedic surgeon who said, "Don't worry about it. It's just a birthmark on the bone. It shouldn't hurt."

I said, "It does hurt."

He was very dismissive of me. I called a friend whose husband was a back surgeon and asked for advice. He pulled some strings and got me in to see an orthopedic oncologist at Mount Sinai. He looked at the bone scan and ordered a biopsy. They called within a few days to say it wasn't cancer, but then called me to come in discuss it further, which was quite unnerving. So it was at that point that they said they had done other tests indicating that I had Erdheim-Chester disease. It's a form of histiocitosis, which itself is rare. But Erdheim-Chester is even rarer. There have only been four or five hundred cases diagnosed worldwide. When I'm presented to residents and interns, Dr. Ho Ping Kong lets them deduce my symptoms, but no one ever guesses what I have. They've never heard of the disease.

The orthopedic oncologist suggested we could remove the bone lesions, but I decided against that, as I did not want to spend six months in a hospital bed. In the end, he sent me to see Dr. Ho Ping Kong. By coincidence, HPK had gone to high school in Jamaica with my ex-husband's father, so I knew he had a soft spot for the family.

When we met, he was very gentle, very caring and forthright in saying he did not know a lot about Erdheim-Chester disease, and that it would be learning process for all of us. He said he would do what he could to find treatment for me, but in the event that he could do nothing, he would be there for me throughout to make sure I was comfortable until the end. That was an experience I had not had before in the medical system, just in terms of humanity. HPK made it clear that I would not be allowed to fall between the cracks. And I've never felt with him that I was falling between the cracks. Sometimes there are very sad things to discuss, but I know I am in good hands. There may be things he has not shared with me yet, but I trust him with that. My daughter, who often comes with me to appointments, said to me, "It's a weird thing, but it's always fun coming here."

It often happens with so-called orphan diseases, for which there is no known drug treatment, that getting funding for off-label use of drugs is very difficult. Kineret costs more than $20,000 a year. It helped for six to seven months, but then stopped working.

At this point, I'm a terminal case, so I'm in palliative care. The pain is tolerable. I rely heavily on a network of friends and hospice groups. I am told that survival is on average 32 months from time of diagnosis, so I'm already into bonus time. I've signed a DNR — do not resuscitate. I've been putting my affairs in order. My daughter will be power of attorney and Dr. Ho Ping Kong talks to her as well. It's not just me that he is taking care of. Before I separated, he looked after my husband as well. He wanted to be sure he was handling my illness.

The whole experience has been almost surreal. I was somewhat lucky to have it diagnosed early, though much of it came down to my gut instinct that something was wrong. And I've had an incredible team to look after me. I spend a lot of time resting, trying to save energy for things I want or need to do — cooking, buying groceries. Some days, all I can do is take a shower, which is very important to me. The pain is unpredictable. I don't drive anymore. I don't sleep well, so I use the iPad to read or email friends or play Scrabble and other games.

But it is what it is.

NO ONE TAKES PLEASURE IN the delivery of bad news. Inevitably, however, there are times — many times — when a physician must play that unenviable role. It is the hardest part of what we do.

My first priority, of course, is to ensure that the facts are indeed correct. Every few years, I hear an account of a patient told that he or she is suffering from an incurable disease. They then bear all the terrible anxiety of that verdict, the tears and depression — only to later be advised that the information was wrong. Someone misread the MRI or CT scan or ultrasound images. Nothing destroys the essential bond of trust between doctor and patient as thoroughly or as fast as a misdiagnosis. So before everything else, I try to ensure that the diagnosis is accurate.

Even a grim diagnosis, however, is not a death sentence. There are interventions to consider, ameliorative treatments if not outright cures, therapies that may minimize symptoms and reduce pain. All of this data must be at your command before you meet the patient.

A cardinal principle applies: you must always speak the truth. However, I sometimes find it easier not to convey all of the truth all at once. Thus, after all the tests are complete, I might use a first session to suggest what the possibilities are, including the worst ones, but then say that I first need to confer with colleagues or review the medical literature, to see what options might be available.

It should be obvious that great sensitivity is required in the telling, though I know of cases where the presentation was heartless, if not cruel. I once treated an elderly woman in Montreal who, a decade earlier, had developed a lump on her breast. The presiding surgeon delivered the news in the worst possible way. "You have breast cancer," he bluntly declared. "And what do we do in these cases?" Then he stood and, reaching toward her with a claw-like hand, made a dramatic sweeping motion. "We cut it off!" When I met her 10 years later, she was still dealing with the trauma of that encounter.

Hopefully, I will have used earlier meetings with patients to prepare them psychologically for a dark outcome. For example, even before I know whether a spot on the lung or a lump on the breast is malignant, I will have told the patient that it could be serious. But I will also suggest that it could be benign. Often, I am asked by the adult children of a patient not to disclose that their aging parent has cancer. I usually agree, but always with the caveat that if I am asked directly by the patient, "Is it cancer?" I will be obliged to answer truthfully. I cannot tell a lie.

The children often fear that their parent may, hearing the prognosis, surrender the will to live. In fact, that almost never happens. The survival instinct is so deeply embedded in the human psyche that despite the pain and suffering, the anxiety and depression, we cling tenaciously to life.

As in so many other medical domains, we are often grappling here with uncertainty. We may not know how far the cancer has advanced or the rate of its metastasis (spread). In turn, we often cannot accurately determine life expectancy. I try to provide the most hopeful assessment that is faithful to the facts as I know them.

I recently had to deliver a diagnosis of acute myeloid leukemia to a patient. Ten years ago, that conversation would have constituted an inescapable death sentence. Today, with advances in stem-cell transplant therapy, the prospects have improved. I consulted the transplant hematologist, who placed the chance of a cure at 30 percent. The chemotherapist (hematologist) gave me better odds of recovery — 64 percent. I considered my patient, an otherwise healthy, symptom-free man of 70, and told him his chances of being cured were 40 percent. I want to give hope, where it is reasonable, but not more hope than is justified by the facts. The patient underwent induction chemotherapy, followed by stem cell transplant. He was doing well 120 days post-transplant.

But at some point, it may be necessary to state unequivocally that the patient has cancer and must consider surgery, chemotherapy or radiation. I then offer my assistance in finding the best possible specialist for what treatment is chosen. And I encourage them to focus on the positive — to do their best to make every day a good day.

If I am asked, "How much time do I have?" I say, "We cannot predict." People may survive for months or years beyond the textbook expectation. Sometimes, in defiance of the odds, the disease arrests itself, or there is a complete reversal.

Certain considerations are obvious. These decisive meetings should be held in private. You must be sure not to be interrupted by phone calls, emails or text messages, and you should avoid looking at your watch. You must allocate as much time as is needed to guide the patient through the discussion, explaining the options. He or she will decide when it is over. At some point, it may be necessary to raise the issue of the estate, which I usually couch in the form of simple questions. "Most people of our age have wills," I say. "Do you have one? Is it up-to-date?"

Generally, I try to meet with the patient alone, unless he or she insists on being accompanied by family members. But it is here again, in this closing chapter of our relationship, that the groundwork laid months or years earlier pays enormous dividends. If you have done a respectable job, you will be able to connect on any number of levels that transcend illness and provide comfort: a discussion of career, of children, of hobbies, of religion, of world affairs, etc. I always know who they are, beyond their status as a patient. Does a human relationship with a caring physician lessen the impact of hearing grave news? I believe it does. I'm neither a surgeon, nor a chemotherapist, but I can be there to help them navigate the system and assure them that I will not abandon them. They take comfort in that assurance.

The late Dr. Robert Buckman, an oncologist, writer and humanist, was perhaps the best physician I ever saw when it came to the delivery of bad news. Highly intelligent, he was also an extraordinary communicator and, in his native England and in Canada — to which he immigrated in 1985 — he worked both as a doctor and as a radio and TV broadcaster. When he arrived here, he had to requalify as a general internist and spent six weeks with me preparing for his exam. He had a genuine knack for dealing with patients facing a grim prognosis. Each approach was different, but he made every patient feel that they were deeply cared for. He later wrote two books on how to render bad news and frequently delivered courses to medical students on the subject.

THE EXPLOSION OF INFORMATION NOW available on the internet has changed the way patients approach and interact with the medical system. As often as not, they now arrive in my office armed with a dossier of symptoms and treatment options for the disease they have self-diagnosed. For the most part, it is better to deal with a well-informed consumer — they are likely to be more proactive about getting better — but there are occasions when their pre-examination research is actually a hindrance. Some are even unable to believe good news, when it is offered.

One 23-year-old young man had developed strange blotches on his skin. Somehow, he became convinced that he had developed leprosy. He had made the rounds of various doctors, all of whom tried to dispel him of his illusion, without success. When I saw him, he arrived with his father, from whom he had been estranged for about 15 years. Somewhere in that complex relationship, I was sure, lay the clue to his misguided self-diagnosis.

"You're my last hope, doctor," he complained when I saw him for the first time.

"Well, let's examine you and see what we can find," I said, neutrally.

We conducted all the necessary tests and soon reconfirmed categorically that he did not, in fact, have leprosy.

"Well, doctor, do I have it?" he asked anxiously at our third meeting.

"No," I said, "you do not have it."

"How do you know?"

"I've seen cases of leprosy," I said. "I've read a lot about it. You have some discolouration, but you have no actual skin changes, no nerve changes and you've had no exposure to other leprosy patients."

I thought I would be conveying joyous news. I was wrong. The young man became abusive, hurling profanities at his father. He had to be dragged out of the office.

I RECALL ANOTHER CASE THAT demonstrates just how tricky it can be to navigate the shoals of the Grey Zone. The patient was Helena, a 78-year-old woman of Greek origin with a significant medical history. Some 12 years earlier, she had had a new mechanical mitral valve implanted, likely for rheumatic heart disease. The surgery had greatly enhanced her quality of life, but now she was complaining of weakness and fatigue. Helena's family doctor had sent her for blood work, which revealed a low hemoglobin count of 100. A second test showed that it was falling — to 90 — clear evidence of anemia. At that point, she was sent to me.

I ordered a number of tests, but was concerned most about one that found occult blood in the stool. We ruled out H. pylori, the common bacteria that causes gastric ulcers, and administered iron. But the hemoglobin level continued to fall, from 90 to 80, then 70 and then 60. Helena had to be anti-coagulated to prevent clotting on the mechanical valve (a standard treatment). She continued to have positive tests for occult blood in the stool. So despite a recent normal exam, we chose to repeat the colonoscopy. This time, the specialist found an ulcer in the cecum, a small pouch-like attachment located at the end of the ileum. The surgeon cauterized it, which stopped the bleeding, and for several months Helena was fine (and very grateful).

Then, a few years ago during the month of October, I learned from her daughter that Helena had been ill, suffering from a 103-degree temperature and chills and feeling disoriented. I saw her the next morning. She was indeed sick, barely able to walk, febrile, tachycardic (a fast pulse) and a little confused. My initial fears focussed on two possibilities. The first was endocarditis, an infection on her mechanical valve. My other thought was West Nile virus. Toronto had experienced a mini epidemic of this mosquito-borne illness some years earlier, which caused several deaths and left many others permanently debilitated. It often presents with features of encephalitis.

"Does your mother do any gardening?" I asked her daughter that morning.

"Why, yes," she said. "She likes to avoid the sun so normally goes out in the morning and evenings."

"And are there many mosquitoes?"

"Oh, yes. Too many. She has even been using mosquito coils in the garden."

We subsequently admitted Helena on the assumption of endocarditis. West Nile, I knew, usually appears in August or September, but because incubation can last as long as three weeks, sometimes in October. So we also ran the West Nile blood test, which came back positive. In the meantime, we ran six separate cultures for endocarditis and they all came back negative. But part of the examination for endocarditis involves an echocardiogram, to check the functioning of the mechanical mitral valve. And on one of these images, we found a 1–2 centimetre mass. What was it — a vegetation on the valve, caused by endocarditis? Or was it a blood clot, caused by the mechanical valve? We didn't know and, short of invasive surgery, we could not answer the question.

Thus did we find ourselves in the Grey Zone, with an identifiable problem but an uncertain treatment approach. So what do you do? If it is endocarditis and you fail to treat it, the patient's life is at risk. She could die in six to eight weeks, or sooner if a staph infection was responsible. Or a piece of the clot, if there is one, could break off, travel to the brain and cause a stroke. Do we administer antibiotics on the assumption that endocarditis is in play? The answer depends on what is best for the patient — this patient, with all her medical history.

In the end, after several days of consultation, the cardiologists and I agreed to treat Helena — with intravenously administered antibiotics — for what we call culture-negative endocarditis, which involved a six-week hospital stay.

Today, Helena has been home for one year and, given her history, is in relative good health. But we still don't know for sure whether our assessment was correct. If you culture negatively for endocarditis — and she did six consecutive times — it's unlikely that you have the condition. But there is something called culture-negative endocarditis — that is, the organism is fastidious and hard to culture.

Even if you make the assumption, the next step is not easy. There's a risk of Clostridium difficile (C-difficile); or pseudo membranous colitis, a potentially lethal condition especially in the elderly; or kidney damage, potential complications of weeks of the antibiotics needed. Her regimen of Coumadin posed another potential complication. Still, for Helena, with the definite mass on the valve, this was the correct decision. My own feeling was that, in addition to the West Nile virus, which is not treatable, the mass was likely a clot on the valve. But because we could not be sure, and because of the dangers of doing nothing — death or disability by endocarditis, the infection itself, a heart condition or stroke — we were effectively forced to administer the six-week antibiotic treatment. It was in the patient's interests.

Grey Zone cases like Helena's — thorny and complex — are more common than you might expect. But they demonstrate again why the art of patient-centred medicine will never entirely go out of fashion.

AN

INTERNIST'S

PERSPECTIVE

Dr. STEPHEN HWANG

Dr. Stephen Hwang earned a master's degree in Public Health (epidemiology) from Harvard School of Public Health, an M.D. from Johns Hopkins University and a B.A. (biochemistry) from Harvard University. His current titles include scientist, Centre for Research on Inner City Health in the Keenan Research Centre of the Li Ka Shing Knowledge Institute at St. Michael's Hospital; director, Division of General Internal Medicine, University of Toronto; associate professor, Department of Medicine, University of Toronto; associate professor, Dalla Lana School of Public Health, University of Toronto; associate professor, Institute of Health Policy, Management and Evaluation, University of Toronto and staff physician, Division of General Internal Medicine, St. Michael's Hospital.

RAISED IN SOUTHERN CALIFORNIA AND educated in the American Northeast, Stephen Hwang came to Canada in the mid-1980s to be closer to his wife's family in Toronto. He had recently graduated from Johns Hopkins with a degree in medicine. His first year in residency was not a happy one. "I realized I wasn't getting the education I had hoped for," he says.

Learning from fellow residents that the city's choice place for training was Toronto Western Hospital (TWH), he made an appointment to see Dr. Herbert Ho Ping Kong, who then directed its residency program.

"I was required to do two years at the same hospital, so I still had one year to go," he recalls. "But I essentially pleaded with him to let me into TWH. He took my pleadings to heart and let me in. I don't know whether he had to pull any strings to do that."

Hwang ended up spending two more years at Western, and

then became chief resident at both Toronto Western and Toronto General. "What I discovered is that Western, led by Ho Ping Kong, had developed an incredible culture of general internists who were expert clinicians and diagnosticians and who took delight in teaching. They showed by example how general internal medicine could be practised and taught. That was a formative experience. At clinics, HPK, as we called him, would grab me and say, 'Look at this patient. Listen to the heart.' Or he'd start grilling me on the sounds made by mitral stenosis, a valve disorder, which is rare now and was uncommon then. I was preparing for my Royal College exams and after I successfully identified mitral stenosis, he said, 'Now I'm confident you'll be okay.'"

For his college exam, Hwang found himself in Montreal's Royal Victoria hospital. At the time, the oral portion of the exam was not standardized. It required physicians to see a real patient, take a full medical history and conduct a full physical examination, and then be grilled by a panel about the findings. "It was a source of dread," Hwang recalls, "because you could encounter a condition you had never seen before, in which case you were probably doomed. Moreover, the patients often seemed to think their role was to withhold information about their condition. So you'd ask, 'Are you short of breath?' And they'd say, 'I'm not sure I'm allowed to tell you.'"

Purely by chance, the patient Hwang encountered for his exam had been attended by Dr. Ho Ping Kong during his years in Montreal. Although she was a lupus sufferer, he had successfully nursed her through pregnancy with the disease. In fact, she was convinced that Ho Ping Kong's treatment had saved both her life and the life of her child.

"So it's not just about skill. HPK is able to form a connection with his patients. They see and feel that his caring is genuine," Hwang says.

Although the number shrinks every year, there are still some conditions, Hwang maintains, that can only be diagnosed by careful physical examination and talking to the patient. "Moreover, as human beings, we require doctors with whom we can form a real connection, not just technicians. You can learn from a teacher that provides the information and facts, but the best teacher is the one who makes a connection with students and inspires them and lights a fire for more learning."

Hwang says he has thought deeply about this issue. "I don't think you can have a fully therapeutic, healing relationship or process if it's purely technical. There are computerized programs that do diagnoses. They were primitive when I was in medical school and they are better now, and I'm sure we will have, perhaps in 10 or 15 years, machines that can do as good a job as the best clinician in making a preliminary diagnosis and ordering the right tests. But I think fundamentally, we would find that unsatisfying and sterile. Very few people would be happy with such a system, even if the right diagnosis was made and the treatment was successful. It's who we are as social beings and why medicine is both a science and art and requires ability to connect with people."

From his own research on public health — he works principally with the disadvantaged and the homeless — Hwang says it's clear that the limiting factors with respect to positive outcomes pertain not to diagnosis and/or treatment but to society's ability to affect the environment of patients and their behaviours.

A case in point is lung cancer. Over the past few decades, medicine has made significant advances in the field, both with respect to surgery and drug therapies. But the fundamental problem remains: how to get people to stop smoking. "We know the answer is not better surgery or chemotherapy," he says. "The answer is to quit smoking. But that's really hard. So it's not a technological problem. It's a human problem."

Many problems in medicine, he insists, are like that. "We could reduce the burden of disease if we spent more time addressing the human contributing factors and less time focussing on better scans or genetic tests. I'm not against technology, but if you look at the untapped potential to reduce disease, the greatest possibilities are in the human area."

Why is it so important to maintain the art of medicine? Without it, Hwang suggests, we will suffer a "loss of common sense. As you become more enmeshed in the technology, you stop listening and seeing what is plainly in front of your face."

Consider, he says, the true story of the British driver so enamoured of his GPS device that he followed its directions blindly — into a river. Unfortunately, in charting the most direct path to the destination, the machine failed to take account of the fact that it followed a road that often washes out in the rainy season.

"In medicine, too," says Hwang, "we sometimes follow the GPS and don't see the river we are about to drive into. With increasing reliance on technology — on the E-patient and lab work — we are losing the skill of looking at the patient and making smart deductions."

The great impediment, he notes, is time. If the art of medicine relies, in the first instance, on getting to know patients and their history, and spending unhurried time in examining them, the reality is that many physicians find their workload an obstacle in the way of that objective.

"We have to be careful," Hwang says, "to create that time for thoughtful contemplation and observation of the patient, including talking to them — despite the constraints and the pressure to move on to the next patient. It requires effort and mindfulness."

One of the "arts," then, is knowing when to invest that time — and when not to. "You can't do every patient, head to toe. You can't take a two-hour history with every patient. Some will require it, but many will not, and you have to be able to identify where and when it will be beneficial and when it will be a waste of time, because the condition or illness does not justify it."

More critically perhaps, with the rise in human longevity, the nature of disease itself is becoming more complex. Increasingly, doctors find themselves treating patients — particularly the elderly — with multiple, chronic illnesses. It's not atypical for a group of internists and specialists to treat a single patient simultaneously for heart failure, diabetes, liver problems, skin cancer and other ailments.

Thus, while modern science has learned how to combat many serious diseases and extended human life, the advance is not without consequences.

Twenty-five years ago, it was unusual to find an elderly patient taking more than five medications a day. Today, says Hwang, "We have medical reconciliation sheets, with space for 12 drugs, and it's not at all uncommon for a single patient to have three sheets." In some ways, he says, "We are victims of our own success."

Our ancestors rarely got cancer because they typically died of infection or trauma before the age of 50. "I don't think we want to go back to the 'good old days,'" Hwang notes, "but the reality is we now have multiple illnesses to treat and we have to decide which ones get priority and set up drug regimens that take account of the complex chemical interactions. It's far more complex than it used to be. We live longer and are healthier — and this is a side effect. It's a reality we have to address."

It's that very element of complexity, he says, that underscores the need for the discipline of general internal medicine. "The specialist knows everything about a narrow area, but a general internist understands the complexity and the big picture. We treat forests, not trees. That role is increasingly needed." The recognition of that may have been lost during the era of subspecialization, but Hwang believes it is coming back.

CHAPTER 9

THINKING
OUTSIDE *the* BOX

Discovery consists in seeing what everyone else has seen and thinking what no one else has thought.

— Albert von Szent-Györgyi, Nobel Prize–winning physiologist

IF PRACTISING THE ART OF medicine is principally about bringing more humanity to the doctor-patient relationship, it is not *only* about humanity. Part of it involves devising creative approaches to diagnosis and treatment, or what I like to call out-of-the-box thinking.

I'm not sure how — or even whether — you can teach future generations of doctors to develop out-of-the-box thinking. The best analogy may be music. You usually need to have years of experience and exposure to the classic forms before you can begin to play jazz. Similarly, in medicine, I would argue that you need to have a broad and deep grasp of basic medicine before you can consider adopting more experimental tactics.

Regardless, it is certainly a skill that physicians young or seasoned would find useful. Quite frequently, disease does not present with the expected or familiar pattern. Especially in an age of multi-system medical problems, disease (and the treatment of it) is becoming a moving target, and physicians need to be agile enough to move with it. I can recall six or seven cases in particular that will help demonstrate what I mean.

Some years ago, the then dean of medicine in Toronto asked me to examine Genevieve, the daughter of a university colleague. Just over 30 years of age, she had long borne the sad burden of neurofibromatosis (NFM), a congenital illness that produces (usually) benign tumours in the brain, spinal cord and other parts of the nervous system.

There is no getting around it: NFM is a nasty disease. These fibrous lesions had already led to a stroke, about a decade earlier, which left Genevieve with partial paralysis. But despite her disability, she was determined to live a normal life. She had earned a certificate in early childhood education, was working part-time in the field and, in her spare time, had managed to become a competent skier.

In addition to the growths on her nervous tissue, Genevieve had developed a large vascular mass — a combination of fibrous tissue and blood vessels — that covered at least half of her trunk. One day, on the ski slopes, she took a nasty spill, falling directly on the vascular mass. She started to bleed profusely. Rushed to Toronto Western Hospital, she had to be administered 35 pints of blood before the bleeding stopped and her equilibrium could be restored. After she was discharged, I was asked to see her.

As if NFM were not enough, she also had an arteriovenous malformation (AVM), an abnormal connection between arteries and veins, likely congenital as well.

I was not a specialist in any of these areas, nor had ever seen this complication of neurofibromatosis before, which I told her. But, after examining her, I did have an out-of-the-box idea that I thought might help. My idea was embolization — a procedure that would implant material, glue or glass particulate, inside the trunk lesion, which would effectively block the flow of blood. If it worked, it was unlikely the mass would bleed again, even in the event of another accident. In fact, if it worked, then the hardened mass might be amenable to removal by a plastic surgeon.

I was on good terms with Dr. Karel Terbrugge, a colleague who had successfully embolized an AV malformation in the brain of another patient of mine, a much more complicated operation. My reasoning was that if Karel could do it in the brain, he should be able to do it on the skin of the torso.

The family agreed to consider it, while I conferred with my colleague about the degree of difficulty involved. Much to my delight, he was extremely optimistic. It took several sittings, but the procedure worked. Later, a surgeon was able to remove about 80 percent of the mass. Some 13 years later, Genevieve has experienced no further problems from that AV malformation.

Where did my idea come? I knew Karel and the success he had previously had in embolizing other AV malformations. I also knew that unless something was done, Genevieve was at risk of hemorrhaging from the massive amount of blood vessels that covered most of her lower trunk. This led me to embolization treatment, with more than satisfactory results.

ON ANOTHER OCCASION, I ATTENDED to Joyce, a 45-year-old British woman of Jamaican heritage, who worked for the civil service. She came to see me with a swollen abdomen and a tentative diagnosis of cirrhosis of the liver, made by her family doctor. I tried to examine her liver and spleen by palpation, but was limited by her pain, which was intense.

I ordered a standard workup, which revealed that her biochemical liver function was normal. Abdominal ultrasound revealed no ascites (excess fluid in the abdomen) and a normal appearing liver. However, a CT scan indicated a blood clot, or thrombosis, in her portal vein, which carries oxygen-depleted

blood from the stomach, the intestines, the spleen, the gallblad-
der and the pancreas to the liver.

Our conclusion was that she was suffering from Budd-Chiari
syndrome, which presents with the precise symptoms that were
affecting Joyce. The ailment, which is extremely rare, is named
after British physician George Budd and Austrian pathologist
Hans Chiari. Uncorrected, it leads to portal vein hypertension,
which can result in fatal hemorrhage from varices (enlarged
blood vessels in the stomach and esophagus). Eventually, we
found the genesis of Joyce's malaise — something called an anti-
phospholipid antibody.

What happens is that the body's immune system manufac-
tures antibodies that attack a type of fat cell — phospholipids.
The damage causes blood clots, like the kind formed in Joyce's
portal vein. That, in turn, gave her the pain, the enlarged spleen,
portal hypertension and varices.

Then Joyce had a transient ischemic attack (TIA), a kind of
mini-stroke. For several hours her arm was paralyzed. The statistics suggest that about 30 percent of people who suffer TIAs
experience a full-blown stroke within a year. Moreover, the TIA
implied that her condition was not confined to the venous system, but also involved her arterial vessels, a potentially more
dangerous situation. She therefore needed preventative therapy
against stroke.

So now, I faced a genuine problem. To treat the underlying portal vein thrombosis, we would typically administer an
anti-coagulation drug, such as warfarin or heparin. The risk, of
course, was that anti-coagulation might precipitate catastrophic
bleeding from her massive esophageal varices.

My proposed solution was again based more on instinct
than hard science. I wrote her a prescription for Ticlid, an anti-
platelet agent. I did not want to use regular anti-coagulation
because of the risks posed by her varices and the strong conse-
quential likelihood of more bleeding. At the same time, some

type of anti-coagulation was clearly needed. I also chose to add a small dose of warfarin (Coumadin), two milligrams daily.

I was honest about the strategy, telling her there were no clear answers for her condition. That was 13 years ago and, apart from a brief stomach ulcer (successfully treated), Joyce has experienced no bleeding from her varices, no further cerebral ischemic attacks (TIA) and no recurrence of her abdominal thrombosis. I can't say definitively that this strategy prevented any of the more nefarious possibilities, but I can say for sure that this unusual combination (dose-wise) provided a good balance between the risks of bleeding versus the danger of thrombosis (clotting).

A PATIENT'S TESTIMONY — *Joyce C.* —————————————

I was raised in Jamaica and England and came to Canada in 1972. I worked for a religious-book publisher for many years and then, for 28 years, with the library and archives department of the federal government. I started to have terrible pains in my stomach in 1985, with swelling, weakness and loss of energy. They treated me for ulcers, but that did not work. I've had pain more or less constantly since then. So many doctors, so many hospitals. Not pleasant. One doctor called me the Mystery Woman. I said, "No, I'm not a mystery. It's that science has yet to figure out a lot of things."

I'd have pain and swelling at work and have to go home. Once, I was hospitalized for three weeks. I woke up one day and found myself bleeding with needles in my arms. I eventually checked myself out of the hospital. The doctors were preparing to do surgery without knowing why. It was hard for me at work. They thought I was lazy or malingering. I had a few CT scans, but they always came back negative. But I knew from the questions they were asking that what I had was serious. Eventually, my family doctor said he had to send me to a specialist. I was supposed to see a liver doctor but she was unavailable, so I ended up with Dr. Ho Ping Kong.

He did a very thorough examination and decided to admit me, to do more tests. After every test, he would come with the result. He'd sit down and explain what was going on. I was more aware than I would otherwise have been, and it's allowed me to avoid the mistakes that other doctors would have made. My portal veins and my spleen were blocked and my liver was in serious condition, though they assured me it could repair itself. There is no known cause, just the effects. That was October 1994. Then I had a relapse and had to be hospitalized again. It felt like my body was on fire. It was as if you could cook a meal on my body. I was in so much pain I could not squeeze the button to call the nurse. I begged the doctors not to touch me, because of the pain.

Then, two years later, I was at a friend's home. I had spent the day picking peas and later that night I could not move. My whole side was numb. Then after daybreak, it started to tingle. I drove to my family doctor. He couldn't believe it because I'd had a stroke. So I went to see Dr. Ho Ping Kong. That's when he started me on these two medications — Coumadin and Ticlid. Since then, I haven't been hospitalized. I have good days and bad days. I tried to go back to work but I couldn't continue. Stress aggravated the condition and it was a stressful job. Dr. Ho Ping Kong advocated for me so that I could work flexible hours. But eventually, it became too much. I was having anxiety attacks. I could not function. I was afraid to get into an elevator. So I took early retirement in 2000. I've been on the same dosage since then. I have no pain today. I'm blessed.

The medical community will lose a vital doctor when HPK retires. I worry who will replace him, for me and for other patients. I was never treated as a number, but as a human being. He listens. He does not push drugs. He is thorough and he takes all measures to find out what is happening before he acts. It would be good if they could all be like him.

IMAGINE A CONDITION SO PAINFUL that it is widely known as the "suicide disease." Such is trigeminal neuralgia (TGN), a neuropathic disorder characterized by acute facial pain. The source of the pain is the trigeminal nerve, the fifth cranial nerve, which branches out to connect with the eye, the ear and the jaw. The actual cause of TGN is unknown. It may be the result of a virus. It may stem from some entrapment or compression of part of the nerve. The truth is, we don't know. What we do know is that its victims suffer bouts of intense pain, which can be triggered by effects as random as a gust of wind or a loud sound.

When I saw Anthony, a business executive, for the first time, he had already been a TGN patient for many years. He had been treated initially with gabapentin, a drug originally designed to deal with epilepsy that has been used with some success for neuropathic pain. Unfortunately, he developed side effects and soon had to suspend usage.

Anthony then sought help from neurosurgeons, who performed what is known as a rhizotomy, a procedure that severs the offending nerves. Like many patients who opt for a surgical solution, his symptoms diminished significantly for a number of years. The benefit, however, was finite. Eventually, the pain returned. A second procedure was then performed — an indication, if nothing else, of how debilitating his condition had become. Unfortunately, it was not nearly as successful.

When I saw him, the pain and its consequent disability were severe. Toronto Western Hospital at the time had only recently acquired a Gamma Knife, a device that allows surgeons to aim beams of radiation on very small targets in the brain. The minimally invasive procedure, known as radiosurgery, was invented by the Swedish neurosurgeon Lars Leksell. It delivers a precise, single dose of ionizing radiation without the standard risks of open neurosurgery. Patients are in and out on the same day and usually back to work the same week.

For years, we and many other hospitals sent patients in need of this operation to Sweden. In 2005, we acquired our own in-house Gamma Knife, mainly to deal with acoustic neuromas — tumours that grow on the nerve that connects the brain and the inner ear. But it can be used for TGN, and Anthony had already been booked for the procedure.

Still, he was uncertain. "What happens if it doesn't work?" he asked me. "What alternatives do I have?"

I had no answer, except that he could not be certain that it would not work. I wasn't at all sure what I could contribute of value. He seemed to be good hands, with both neurologists and neurosurgeons. But in the course of conversation, I asked him if anyone had prescribed for him the drug Lyrica, the trade name for an anticonvulsant remedy known as pregabalin. No one had.

Would he be willing to try it, I asked, before committing to radiation via the Gamma Knife? He would.

So I put him on 50 milligrams of Lyrica, once a day, about a third of the usual dose. When he returned, six weeks later, the pain was dramatically reduced — registering a one on a scale of 10, he told me. And his wife even credited me with saving the marriage. Four years later, he is largely pain free. That said, it is still possible that its efficacy will fade with time, and he may yet become a candidate for Gamma Knife surgery. In addition, Anthony will soon need a kidney transplant. He donated one of his kidneys some years ago and, now a diabetic, can no longer function with just one.

A PATIENT'S TESTIMONY — *Anthony D.* ─────────
I am 65 years old. I was born in Shanghai and came to
Canada at age two. I'm half Portuguese, half English, with
some Chinese mixed in there as well. My father was a general practitioner so I had some knowledge of the medical
system and how to navigate it, which was ultimately very
helpful. I have a master's degree in social work and have
run a charitable organization for children for 20 years.

My problem began about 20 years ago. I was having
some root canal work done and experienced intense pain
in my jaw. My dentist thought the problem was a specific
tooth, so he took it out. The pain continued and actually
worsened. Then he thought it was another tooth and took
that out. In the end, they removed three teeth and I underwent two root canals procedures. I was still in great pain.

I finally got on the right medical track and was diagnosed with trigeminal neuralgia. It's a strange disease. The
nerves near the eye go out of control and shoot out pain
signals uncontrollably, like electric shocks. Sometimes,
the pain is annoying and sometimes it is totally disabling.
No common pain relievers touch it, and weird things trig-
ger it, like wind or even walking. I had a job at that time
that required me to speak in front of large groups and I
never knew day to day if I could function. But I did. I
sucked it up.

Neurologists prescribed some stronger medications,
but I was allergic to both of them. Then I saw a neurosurgeon and he eventually performed a rhizotomy, which zaps
the nerve. It was high risk, but I felt I had no choice. If they
missed the precise spot, I'd have lost muscle control of the
eye — unable to blink or walk around with a droop. The
surgery worked, but I was left totally numb on that side of
the face. You could slap me and I wouldn't have known it.

They told me I should be okay for 10 years, but then the

nerve would likely regenerate and they were right. The pain returned. I'd have raging attacks — white light pain — during which I could not open my eyes. I'd sit in a dark room in complete silence waiting for it to pass. I tried meditation techniques and, while they mitigated the pain, they just touched the edge of it. I tried acupuncture, which worked as long as I was lying on the table. But the pain returned immediately afterward. I slept with a mouth guard — no difference.

So I went back to the neurosurgeon, who was about to retire. I asked him whether he could repeat the procedure. "Oh," he said, "we don't do that anymore. That's barbaric. What we do now is pack a gel on the nerve."

"Okay," I said, "can you do that?"

They tried it and it did nothing. He then sent me to Toronto Western, where they were doing the new Gamma Knife surgery. I was not enthusiastic. They cut into the back of your skull. It works in only two out of three cases. And the effects only last for two years. It was at that point that friends sent me to Dr. Ho Ping Kong, who they called a healer. He examined me and reviewed the various drugs I've tried, without effect. He said, "Have you tried Lyrica?"

"No."

"Well," he said, "it's usually the seventh choice, but if you haven't tried it, what do you have to lose?"

Instant relief. I mean, instant. And no side effects. Because other drugs worked by killing me. I'd fall asleep driving my car. I felt out of control. This drug, Lyrica — once a day, easy. That was four years ago. About every four months, I feel the nerve getting cranky. But the drug blocks the signal. Otherwise, I've been fine. It's amazing to me, because I'd been seeing the top doctors, the top neurologists, the best scientists, who were going down a whole other path. I'd been mangled by dentists and lived through 15 years of hell. It has had a profound impact on my life, and I was looking at severe solutions. The solution should have been found way upstream. But that is the mystery of medicine. The other doctors are not idiots. They are well informed and well intentioned. But it isn't about science. It's about art, which Ho Ping Kong pays attention to. I now tease him and call him the Great Healer.

MOST OF THE PATIENTS I SEE are sent by specialist or subspecialist colleagues in the Toronto hospital community. Occasionally, however, I agree to review a case that comes from a general practitioner. Such was the origin of my involvement with Phong, a 37-year-old man Vietnamese man. Six years earlier, Phong had been shot in the stomach by armed men, attempting to rob his computer hardware store. As a result, he lost his spleen, parts of his liver and intestine and suffered damage to his kidney. It was a terrible episode, but he did recover.

A few weeks before I saw him, suffering from urinary frequency and feeling unwell, he went to his local hospital's emergency department. They prescribed a week-long course of antibiotics and sent him home. A week later, he returned, feeling worse. He now complained of insomnia and severe backache. Again, he was given a prescription for antibiotics and again sent home. However, the hospital did organize a CT scan, which proved normal.

Another week passed, and Phong continued to deteriorate. At this point, he visited his family doctor. The pain, he reported, was 10 on a scale of 10 and had begun to radiate into his testicles. Blood work showed a platelet count of almost a million (versus a norm of 400,000), anemia, a sedimentation rate over 100 (compared to a normal level of under 15) and a C-reactive protein reading of 150 (versus a norm of 10–12).

Six weeks had passed from onset to the time that appeared in my office. The poor man was in agony. "This is worse than being shot," he told me.

Our working hypothesis was that it was prostatitis, an inflammation of the prostate, and we continued to keep Phong on Cipro, hoping that after six weeks, the drug would finally kill the bacteria. But I was not at ease with the working diagnosis. There were some symptoms of prostatitis that he did not have, and the intense pain in the lower back suggested that something else was going on. My instinct was that the persistent prostatitis could have led to Reiter's syndrome, an arthritic condition that could eventually lead to sacroiliitis.

It took about 10 days, but I arranged an MRI, which showed that he had osteomyelitis of lumbar-sacral spine, a potentially lethal illness. The disc becomes infected and inflamed; in time, the infection can literally eat away your spine. We tried to drain it with a needle, but the cultures proved negative, so we could not actually prove our diagnosis. We knew, of course, that he could still be infected, despite the antibiotics and the normal CT scan.

Nevertheless, we felt confident that we had identified the genesis of his problem and promptly put him on another six-week course of intravenous antibiotics. Without that intervention, Phong could have been a paraplegic in three weeks. Slowly, he improved. We also sent him for a series of immunization shots (pneumococcus, meningococcus, Haemophilus). What we should have realized sooner is that, with his spleen removed, he was vulnerable to invasion by encapsulated and other organisms. Still, by thinking outside the box, I'm quite sure that we literally saved his life.

PHONG'S SPLEEN REMINDS ME OF another instructive out-of-the-box dossier. For almost 30 years, I or a senior colleague has presided over Morning Report — an 8 a.m. session during which a designated medical intern or resident presents a new patient case, from the previous night's inventory in the emergency department. The challenge for those assembled is to use the details of the case to make the right diagnosis. The tacit competition yielded some very lively discussions.

When I chair the meeting, I typically adopt a form of the Socratic method that I learned many decades ago at my Jesuit college in Jamaica. I provide cryptic clues about the case under discussion — clues often drawn from the morning news, weather and occasionally sports reports. Successive waves of medical students and residents have learned that, to prepare for my appearances, they would be well advised to familiarize themselves with current events. My goal is not simply to enliven the proceedings, but to make the learning interactive and more memorable.

On one particular morning, one of the residents told us about Josh, a 22-year-old second-year medical student and hockey player at the University of Toronto. The previous weekend, the University of Toronto team had travelled to Quebec City to play against Université Laval. That involved two 12-hour bus rides, interrupted only by the game, a meal and a short night's sleep. During the game, Josh was crushed into the boards, but not seriously hurt.

Nevertheless, soon after returning home, he was feeling enough pain in the left part of his chest to visit the emergency department. He reported that it hurt to take a deep breath and he also had a sore throat. The first instinct of the attending staff was that, because of his long bus ride and perhaps somewhat dehydrated because of the hockey game, this was likely a pulmonary embolism — a blood clot in the lung. So they immediately administered the blood thinner heparin.

"But he's a healthy young man," I told the Morning Report. "There was no fracture. So, despite the long bus ride, how likely is it that he'd develop a pulmonary embolism? What else might it be? What else is there in that region, structurally?"

"The spleen," someone said.

"So could it be a ruptured spleen? What would rupture the spleen?"

"The injury during the game," came the answer. "Being pushed against the boards."

"But the injury was minor," I reminded them. "Who else gets a ruptured spleen?"

"People with leukemia," one resident suggested.

"That's correct. And if you have leukemia, you are frequently what?" No one had the answer, so I provided it. "You are thrombocytopenic," meaning that you are deficient in blood platelets and prone to bleeding.

"But again, he's otherwise healthy, with no other symptoms," I said. "Any other suggestions?"

"Mononucleosis."

"Aha," I said. "And what happens to the spleen then?"

"It gets larger and softer and it may rupture."

"What else might suggest mononucleosis?"

"The sore throat."

"Very good. So we have put him on heparin to promote bleeding when, in fact, if he has mononucleosis and a ruptured spleen, he is already bleeding. He could bleed to death."

Needless to say, this reversal of the verdict already arrived at provoked some concern. A CT scan and ultrasound were quickly arranged, which confirmed the ruptured spleen. Blood tests later verified mononucleosis.

You might think there should have been more evidence of bleeding, but this is where anatomical and pathological knowledge is critical. The spleen may rupture into the peritoneal cavity and produce massive volume depletion, shock and abdominal pain — obvious signs of bleeding. But the patient may also experience what we call a subcapsular hemorrhage, where the blood is contained, at least temporarily, by a fibrous covering; it may rupture later — or not. In the first instance, an emergency splenectomy — removal of the spleen — would be needed. Fortunately, the latter was what occurred with Josh. We immediately stopped the heparin and watched him carefully for the next several days. He soon recovered.

ONE DAY ABOUT FOUR YEARS ago, I had a telephone call from Paul, a successful businessman in his mid-60s and a longtime patient of mine. He'd had some heart issues a decade earlier and, even before all the evidentiary studies about statins were in, I had started him on a course of these cholesterol-reducing drugs. When he called, Paul was on business in Florida. He'd being exercising, he said, and had experienced some angina-like chest pain.

"I had it just after I started, but then it disappeared," he said. "I worked through it. I did my usual five kilometres on the treadmill."

This is a familiar condition to cardiologists — so-called walk-through angina. If the heart makes a gradual adaptation to the increased stress of exercise, the pain subsides. The common assumption is that this condition constitutes so-called stable angina — nothing to worry about immediately. If the pain does not abate, then it is labelled unstable angina, and the patient is likely a candidate for a battery of tests, including, if necessary, an angiogram.

Paul was looking for reassurance that nothing serious was wrong. "I asked some doctors here and they said it's probably fine. What do you think?"

My response was instinctive. "I don't think it's okay. When are you coming home?"

"Tonight."

"I'm going to see how soon we can get you an appointment with a cardiologist. I'll call you back in 10 minutes."

At 8 a.m. the next morning, Paul was given a stress test at Toronto General Hospital. At 8:30, he went into the angio suite to have an angiogram. A few hours later, I received a call from his brother-in-law, a doctor, thanking me. The procedure had found a significant arterial blockage. Angioplasty — a balloon stent — had been performed.

Symptoms of angina are often difficult to read. Heart pain can be a great mimic. It can manifest itself as an upset stomach, as heartburn, as nausea, as a pain in the jaw, as profuse sweating, even on occasion as an acute pain in the thumb — and nothing more. Sometimes, angina comes on in the wee hours of the morning — 3 or 4 a.m. — though we aren't sure why. Perhaps 70 percent of the time, it presents with the classic symptoms of squeezing and pressure in the chest, with a feeling of impending doom. But about a third of the time it takes other forms.

It would have been easy for me to assume, as the doctors Paul consulted in Florida had, that he was basically fine, because he had managed to work through the initial treadmill pain. My instinct — my willingness to think outside the box — told me this might be serious. I'm delighted to report that because of his stents, Paul has been free of angina-like pain ever since.

BY NOW, IT IS PROBABLY CLEAR that many diseases fall into the challenging realm of I-can't-prove-you-have-it-and-you-can't-prove-you-don't. The only way to treat the illness is to devise a therapeutic trial for a single patient, testing various medications until we find one that effectively eliminates or reduces the symptoms. Even then, of course, we never know definitively whether we have relieved or cured the ailment we suspected. But we know something more important — that we have helped the patient resume a normal life.

The abdominal migraine — an offshoot of the classic migraine headache — is one of these problematic conditions. It is neither rare nor common. The medical literature suggests that it is a phenomenon principally seen in children, but that has not been my experience. Every few years, I meet an adult patient who has its symptoms — abdominal pain, nausea and lethargy. The first step is to determine if anything more serious might be involved.

Not long ago, I treated Sonya, a 35-year-old Hungarian woman, who had been referred by her family physician. She had been unwell for about six months, complaining of non-specific nausea and fatigue. The condition had begun to impinge on her normally active lifestyle.

I ordered a limited workup to check for anemia or peptic ulcer. These proved negative, as had an endoscopy — a probe of the upper gastrointestinal tract — arranged earlier. I also determined that Sonya had no kidney or brain disease. But when I took her history, she allowed that she had in the past experienced classical migraines with flashing lights and sensitivity to noise. I explained that it was possible her migraine was affecting her stomach, and that I wanted to prescribe a beta blocker, propranolol. Beta blockers are more commonly used to treat cardiac patients, but a small dose of 10 milligrams twice daily has also been shown to be preventative of migraine. Three months later, she returned, with no signs of nausea. Again, I could not prove my diagnosis was correct, but she was clearly improved — and has remained so — without exposing her to invasive tests, significant risk or medications with more pernicious side effects.

Dr. ANGELA CHEUNG

Dr. Angela Cheung is a senior clinician scientist at the Toronto General Research Institute (TGRI), investigating osteoporosis and post-menopausal health problems, as well as a professor of Medicine at the University of Toronto and a practising general internist.

THE DAUGHTER OF A HONG KONG PEDIATRICIAN, Angela Cheung's introduction to medicine was made for her even before her teens. Helping out in her father's office, she found herself calling parents to give them advice on how to treat their sick children.

She did an undergraduate degree in physics at Bryn Mawr College and her medical degree at Johns Hopkins University. By then, her family had relocated from Hong Kong to Toronto, a fortuitous development that, later, allowed her to immigrate to Canada as a physician under family reunification policies.

At Johns Hopkins, Cheung debated between choosing internal medicine or pediatrics, but ultimately decided her "personality was not cut out for family medicine. I want depth. I need to know more. I enjoyed internal medicine more than pediatrics. It was easier and more satisfying to deal with adults."

In Toronto, Cheung did a three-year residency, then a fourth year in general internal medicine — at the time, one of only three such residents in all of Toronto. Again, she wrestled with the next decision — this time between the conflicting tugs of clinical practice and research. "I didn't want to give up on either. It was the bane of my work life. I had to choose, but was on the fence. So I went away to Harvard to do a four-year Ph.D., with a thesis on post-menopausal health."

She returned to Toronto four years later as junior staff, one of only two women practising general internal medicine. There are still few women in the field. Cheung says she is the first woman to attain a professorship while climbing through the ranks as an academic general internist.

"It was a stressful period. I had just had a baby and, at the time, you were expected to effectively earn your salary by writing and winning research grant proposals."

Cheung had been exposed to Dr. Herbert Ho Ping Kong as a medical resident and had admired his humane and caring approach — not only to patients but to his team of doctors. "He does have a human touch and he does care how his mentees are doing. I remember when I was on junior staff at the Toronto General and he was at the Western, he made a special trip here to see how I was doing. That made an impression on me. He wanted to assure me that things would be okay. It did help lift my spirits. He's been a mentor to me. If he sees something, he points the way." The problem, she says, is that there are very few clinicians of HPK's calibre.

Coming to Canada from the United States, Cheung says she noticed that she was more proficient in doing medical procedures, such as taps and punctures. "So I was fairly efficient in looking after patients." But she was less skilled, she found, in being able to distinguish between types of heart murmurs. "When I came as a first-year resident, there were various murmurs I had never even heard." Now, when she teaches her own students, she not only uses Harvey — the University Health Network's murmur simulator — but also takes them to patient bedsides to hear the real thing, "because there is variation. Everyone is different."

Cheung takes a measured approach to the rise of technology in medicine. "It can put a distance between patient and doctor," she says. "But it can also make things easier and improve things. You can use technology to help care for the patient, but you can also miss the point, by concentrating on the technology and not the patient. Then it becomes a problem."

Although the proliferation of medical knowledge has spurred specialization and subspecialization, Cheung is optimistic that internal medicine — the role of the academic generalist — will not soon fade away. If anything, it will become more important.

But other changes are likely. Cheung sits on an international committee now examining the future of health policy. Some procedures, she concedes — laser eye surgery, for example — simply don't require the level of education now demanded. "Do we really need someone to have gone through four years of medical school, four years of residency and another three years of specialization to carry out a relatively simple procedure that a high-school student with good hand-eye coordination could perform?" she asks. "Do we really need that kind of vigorous training, which requires people to rack up huge debts and then charge a thousand dollars to help pay off the debt?"

Similarly, she asks, if you go for a colonoscopy, you obviously want it done by an experienced specialist for whom the procedure is routine, someone who will know what to look for. But do we need someone who has 12 to 15 years of training to do a colonoscopy? "Health care costs are becoming a larger portion of the GDP and can we afford it?" Medicine needs to be rational, she maintains. "Why should someone who intends to do laser eye surgery have to do a rotation in orthopedic surgery? You learn a lot of things in medical school that you don't actually retain."

What medical schools need to do a better of job of teaching, she says, are the soft skills. "Yes, you need to know how to put in a line, because if you do it wrong, you puncture a lung. But you also need to know how to break bad news, how to sit with patients and discuss a mistake that might have been made, how to listen, how to be a comfort. It's TLC. Sometimes, I tell my students, 'You have to just let the patient speak or vent. Don't sit at the nurse's station and just concentrate on the numbers from their tests and forget about the patient.' That's really crucial. Our job is to look after patients, not numbers."

A

CARDIOLOGIST'S

PERSPECTIVE

Dr. MATTHEW SIBBALD

Dr. Matthew Sibbald is an award-winning clinical teacher at
the University of Toronto and an interventional cardiologist at
Toronto's University Health Network. He did his residency at
the University of Toronto, was named chief resident and later
completed both his M.A. and Ph.D. in medical education at the
University of Maastricht in the Netherlands.

LIKE MANY OF THE EMERGING medical superstars now gathered
around Toronto Western Hospital's Centre for Excellence in
Education and Practice (CEEP), Dr. Matthew Sibbald had his first
introduction to Dr. Herbert Ho Ping Kong in medical school.

The way it typically works, Sibbald explains, is that students
spend the first two years in the classroom and then, during the
next two years, graduate to clerkships, shadowing residents and
interns. "It's an eye-opening time," he says, "because you are
really seeing patients and the inside of hospital for the first time.
It can be overwhelming."

His introduction was Morning Report, a Socratic teaching session attended by doctors, interns, residents and clerks.
"Herbert often led it, and you discuss a patient's case. But he
would lead you to the diagnosis by means of these very strange
verbal clues. What the heck is going on? I was totally mystified."

Among students, there was a culture of trying to prepare for
these morning sessions, by sharing often-used clues on the shuttle bus between hospitals. "'Howling at the moon' was used to
incite a diagnosis of lupus," Sibbald remembers. "I think what he
was trying to do was to get people primed and ready to jump to
these subtleties, so that these things would come to mind when
faced with difficult cases."

Later, Sibbald followed Ho Ping Kong as he treated patients in a clinic setting. "He often found some very unusual things. I remember one gentleman who had been unwell for months, losing weight and sweating and feeling deeply fatigued. He'd been sent from his GP to an internist, who had done an elaborate series of tests, which proved inconclusive.

"HPK found a prominent heart murmur," Sibbald recalls, "which led to some blood cultures and, ultimately, a diagnosis of endocarditis on his aortic valve. He had surgery in rather short order. In clinic, there were multiple signs that this diagnosis was in play, but they were all individually subtle and easily passed over. The murmur was the sentinel piece and, at that point in my training, I don't think I fully appreciated the severity of the diagnosis or the difficulty in making it."

The subtleties included finding a slightly enlarged spleen, "not something everyone would routinely look for or, if they did, focussing on that abnormality and connecting it to other things," Sibbald says. "Another one was tiny hemorrhages under the nail beds — so-called splinter hemorrhages in the hands and/or feet. That, again, might not be noticed or, if noticed, not considered germane. But in the cluster of a very sick person and an enlarged spleen, it is something to consider."

Another distinguishing feature of these clinics was the extraordinary range of rare and difficult cases that Ho Ping Kong was called on to diagnose. In most clinics, clerks were exposed to generalized, not very serious problems for which the solution was relatively predictable. "Even at the specialist level," Sibbald says, "much of medicine is about reassurance and basic testing around common diseases. Those rules did not apply in his clinics. It was always fascinating."

Ho Ping Kong was particularly strong, he says, with finding variations on vasculitis, which is an inflammation of the blood vessels that can present in many different and unusual ways. "A disease that is at once rare and presents in unusual ways can be very difficult to diagnose. Much depends on the size of the blood vessels afflicted and the patterns. When the medium-sized vessels are inflamed, people get very sick, with accompanying weight loss. But there is no blood work you can do to verify it. Even a blood indicia of inflammation, like a sedimentation rate, doesn't give you the diagnosis. You need an experienced clinician who has seen it before. Or you need specialized imaging which, when I was resident, was not routinely available. I learned a lot from him about these illnesses. I remember a case arriving by ambulance from another hospital, where they could not make the diagnosis . . . He took one look at the patient and said, 'I know what this — it's polyarteritis. You need prednisone.' And the residents would just look at each other with astonishment. How is it possible to walk into a room and see someone for the first time and in three minutes make the diagnosis with so little other corroborating data? And the answer is pattern recognition — he's seen it before and he remembers what to look for."

After his clinics, Sibbald recalls running home to his textbooks to find more information on exotic diseases and medical terms he heard Ho Pong Kong routinely discuss. Only with time and more exposure did "I grasp how warm and disarming he can be," says Sibbald. "He sees the whole person, not just a patient. They become really attached to him and the attraction is personal."

The challenge faced by medical schools trying to model that kind of humane practice is enormous, he allows. "I do think it's a teachable entity, although few trainees," Sibbald observes, "express much interest in learning how to engage patients or navigate a system. They want to learn about specific diseases or a group of diseases. But the other has to be role modelled for them, perhaps by taking trainees aside after they've examined a patient and asking, 'Why do you think that didn't go as well as it might have?'"

"Learning medicine is like putting up a scaffold to organize what is just a sea of information," he says. "A lot of it is very structured and hard to apply. Herbert's way of teaching is very different. It comes from his experience and is very much centred on the art, trying to connect the dots, and it's practically helpful."

The diagnostic charts taught in lectures or in textbooks tend to be clustered around pathologic entities — a group of diseases that all connect pathologically, Sibbald explains. "You can have all that information in your head, but when you walk into a room with a patient, it doesn't necessarily come out. So what HPK does is reorganize that information for trainees, to make it useful in real-life terms."

One of Sibbald's own research interests is in documenting how doctors reorganize knowledge, making the transition from book learning to practical learning, and showing how experts do it. "I think what makes an expert is not the facts that they know, but how they organize them, both with patients and with medical information. And facts change. You have to build your own functional knowledge base. But like most skills, it needs to be practised. Less time in the classroom, perhaps, and more with patients, particularly because most medical students will already have spent three or four years in lecture theatres acquiring scholarly, scientific knowledge in biology, chemistry and anatomy and physics. What's learned in the classroom can be applied well in the classroom, but poorly outside of it. When you have to struggle with a clinical problem, trying to determine what information is valuable, that's a much more useful task than having a lecturer tell you how the world is organized."

The emphasis laid on the sciences as prerequisites for medicine, Sibbald argues, may tailor the dominant character that emerges. To advance the art of medical practice, he suggests, more emphasis likely needs to be put on teaching the humanities — history, philosophy and the softer social sciences. "These are intellectually expanding domains for people on their own professional journey and helpful ways of looking at the world and life. By exposing students to other streams of knowledge, they may begin to see the possibilities of learning in other places. It's not a major focus in Canadian medical schools."

Sibbald credits Ho Ping Kong with being both an advocate and a mentor for his research interests. "He encouraged me. He told me what I needed to do if I wanted to go the route I have. He found me a way to fund it and organize it, while sheltering me from political forces within the institution, and still allowing me to be connected to patients and to the clinic."

In 2011, Sibbald earned a master's degree in Health Professions Education from the University of Maastricht in the Netherlands, and in 2013 completed his Ph.D. there as well. His thesis was entitled *Is that Your Final Answer? How Doctors Should Check Decisions.* "I think psychology has something to say about how we make decisions and when we need to pause," he says. "We all live with uncertainty, but we can't be incapacitated by it. We still have to act and we learn a lot from our mistakes. Having a culture in which we can talk about them is healthy."

CHAPTER 10

Of FEVERS,
EPIDEMICS *and*
EPIDEMIOLOGY

*The work of epidemiology is related to unanswered questions,
but also to unquestioned answers.*

— Dr. Patricia Butler

MEDICAL EDUCATION HAS CHANGED DRAMATICALLY during the
last half century. In the vanguard of these changes was Canada's
Mcmaster University Medical School in Hamilton. Under the
leadership of cardiologist John Evans, who became its founding
dean, internal medicine specialist Bill Spaulding, respirologist
E.J. Moran Campbell, and medical educators Howard Barrows
and Geoff Norman, McMaster — beginning in 1965 — dramatically reshaped the curriculum, de-emphasizing the traditional
approach to academic lectures and formal examinations.

Instead, it created a radically new model, based on self-
directed study, creative thinking and problem-based learning.
The system proved so successful that universities all over the
continent began to emulate it, including the prestigious Harvard
Medical School, which called its own program New Pathway.

They might well have added an asterisk to that title; it was new when McMaster pioneered the concept.

An important part of the McMaster philosophy was to admit a broader range of applicants to its medical school than had previously been the norm. Thus, students with arts, philosophy or political science backgrounds — or people who had been out of school and working for some years — stood as good a chance of winning a coveted slot as recent physics and chemistry graduates. And while grades continued to be important, McMaster placed a premium on other life experience, including extracurricular activities, travel and volunteer work in the community.

My own feeling is that one's background is less important than one's character. And character is more important than curriculum. If you pick the best people and if they have the right intentions, and if they are well led by experienced physicians, you will turn out some very fine doctors. An awful lot of learning has nothing to do with textbooks or formal lectures. It's what you metaphorically absorb, osmotically, in living at the hospital and breathing the air of medicine, day after day.

When you put on the doctor's white coat, you don't leave one self behind and become a new self. You bring it all with you, your personality, your ideas, your idiosyncrasies, for better or worse. And in our increasingly globalized world, the better read, travelled and exposed to other cultures you are, the better a doctor you are likely to make.

I spent many years, both at McGill and the University of Toronto, sitting on panels of admission and interviewing prospective medical students. Of course, the applicants we accepted displayed a broad range of academic intelligence and personality traits. But only rarely did we admit someone with whom we later felt we had made a clear mistake.

I recall one particular example — a young man who consistently displayed what can only be called an egregious bedside manner. I witnessed his combination of arrogance and callousness on several occasions. The worst instance involved his treatment of an elderly heart patient.

"You have severe angina caused by atherosclerosis, by your reckless eating and drinking habits," he told him bluntly. "You could die of it!"

The stress of that exchange caused the man — who did not drink and was slim — to suffer a heart attack within minutes.

Later, I failed the student, for this and other misdemeanors. The truth is, I was failing him for lack of good character — the sine qua non of what we do. He was just not the sort of person likely to bring credit to the profession. The more I saw of his behaviour, the more certain I became that he did not belong.

He appealed the decision and used some influence to have himself reinstated. Then, he foolishly made a personal long-distance call to the United States and billed it to the hospital. When confronted, he at first denied it and then tried to blame the hospital call centre operators. In what became the last straw, he took out his anger on the operators by finding an axe and physically destroying part of their offices. That, thankfully, was the last straw — and the end of his medical career.

MCMASTER'S FIRST CHAIR OF MEDICINE was Moran Campbell, a brilliant respirologist who did groundbreaking research on so-called smoker's disease — chronic obstructive pulmonary disease (COPD). While at London's Hammersmith Hospital, Campbell observed that patients admitted to hospital with this illness often died, while those who stayed home survived. The reason: the hospital patients had been given too much oxygen, which was effectively a poison because it suppressed their respiratory drive.

McMaster's broader program in clinical epidemiology was led by another brilliant physician, David Sackett, an American who established it as a real modern science. Out of this program came a generation of A-list researchers that made major strides in a variety of topic areas and thought deeply about measurement and biostatistics in medical practice. The program promoted and elevated evidence-based medicine, which changed the fundamental ways of medical practice and, indeed, of medical education. To this day, it remains a leader in the field. Sackett wrote two enduring medical textbooks and later established the Oxford Centre for Evidence-Based Medicine in the U.K.

Another McMaster star was Jack Hirsh, an Australian-born hematologist. In one of several research breakthroughs, he assisted Henry Barnett of University Hospital in London, Ontario, in establishing once-lowly aspirin as a treatment of choice in the prevention of heart attack and stroke. Hirsh almost singlehandedly rewrote the principles of diagnosis and treatment of deep vein thrombosis and pulmonary embolism.

In the United States, the rise of evidence-based medicine was championed by epidemiologist Alvan Feinstein at Yale University. Indeed, he coined the phrase clinical epidemiology, which became one of key foundation stones of modern medical practice.

In fairness, both Sackett and Feinstein were building on the innovations of British physician Sir Austin Bradford Hill, who led the groundbreaking post-war study that, for the first time, established the indisputable link between lung cancer and cigarette smoking. Sadly, it took another 30 years — and untold millions of lung cancer deaths — before the U.S. government, under the aegis of the Surgeon-General, acknowledged the truth.

Another landmark study involved fever of unknown origin (FUO), published by physicians Robert Petersdorf and Paul Beeson in 1961. Between 1952 and 1958, the two researchers studied 100 consecutive patients with FUO in Baltimore, and concluded that they broke down into various categories: infections (36 percent); malignancies (19 percent); inflammatory or rheumatologic diseases (15 percent); miscellaneous (23 percent) and undiagnosed (including malingering, 7 percent).

Five decades later, the same rough distribution applies, although infections tend to be more common (40–60 percent) in tropical and subtropical countries. Petersdorf and Beeson defined fever of unknown origin as being anything above 38.3 degrees Celsius for more than three weeks, with the patient in hospital for at least one week. Nowadays, we substitute a week of outpatient investigation for the hospital stays, which have declined dramatically. This study had a major influence on my own generation and gave us some reliable diagnostic benchmarks for approaching FUO, a relatively common and difficult diagnostic entity, with potential for serious illness.

I WAS ONCE ASKED TO examine Colin, a young aircraft engineer of 30 who had suddenly gone deaf in both ears. The assumption was that his long hours of environmental exposure in an aircraft assembly plant had caused the condition. But he had other serious problems, including fever of unknown origin, accompanied by chills, weight loss and anemia.

He arrived at my office with his wife and parents, who were clearly concerned.

"You've got to do something, doctor," his wife said, "or he's going to die. We have three young children."

I assured her I would do the best I could, but would need perhaps a week or 10 days to carry out some investigations. In the meantime, I told them, "It may be necessary to have you readmitted to hospital here."

Then his mother interjected sharply. "We're not going back there. I am fighting all the time with the nurses and doctors on the ward." At that point, she removed a piece of paper from her pocket and started to recite a litany of complaints about how insensitive staff had been to her son's condition. I detected the hint of a Scottish accent as she spoke and sensed a more than common knowledge of medical issues.

"By any chance," I said, "are you a nurse or a doctor?"

"I'm a nurse," she conceded.

"And might you be from Scotland, perhaps Edinburgh?"

"How did you know that?"

"And did you work at Edinburgh Western General Hospital?"

"Yes," she said.

"Well, I was there in 1970," I said. I then rattled off the names of several doctors I had worked with, people she had known.

With that, she almost started to cry. She promptly took her paper, folded it up and put it away.

"Doctor," she said, "just do whatever you need to do."

I was subsequently able to determine that Colin was suffering from polyarteritis nodosa, an autoimmune disorder — a form of vasculitis — that inflames the organs, joints and large blood vessels. His deafness had not, in fact, been caused by environmental exposure, but by something known as mononeuritis multiplex — damage to the nerves in both ears, caused by vasculitis of the vessels supplying blood to the auditory nerves. We started him on a course of high-dose prednisone, which led to recovery from his severe systemic illness.

AMONG THE OTHER CASES IN my own dossier, one of the most interesting involved fever of unknown origin. The patient was referred to me by a former student, Dr. Ophyr Mourad, now an accomplished internist working at another hospital and an award-winning teacher. In fact, Dr. Mourad had co-authored a scholarly paper on FUO. He had been seeing Serge, a Quebec-born businessman in his 40s, for almost three years and, though Dr. Mourad had conducted all the right tests, had been unable to identify the cause of the fever.

Serge was seriously debilitated, losing weight and his ability to concentrate. His condition had effectively forced him to retire, since he no longer trusted himself to handle complex financial transactions. These periods of fogginess, as we subsequently learned, may have indicated the formation of protein deposits — amyloidosis — in the brain. But more of this later.

I repeated a number of the tests Dr. Mourad had performed, without new results. The tincture of time did not help. Time passed and Serge showed no improvement. Every month he was experiencing fevers of 39 and 40 degrees Celsius.

I asked him to keep a detailed record of his fevers, how long they lasted and the temperature. At the time, I wondered whether he might have Pel-Ebstein disease, a rare condition in which the fever spikes for four or five days every six weeks. But Pel-Ebstein is commonly associated with Hodgkin's lymphoma and Serge's fevers did not follow that pattern and there was no evidence of lymphoma.

I also considered familial Mediterranean fever (FMF), so-called because it typically strikes people whose genetic background is in the Middle East and North Africa — Armenians, Arabs, Turks and Jews. But there were no such links on either side of Serge's family tree — only French Catholics, for several generations — so we ruled it out clinically.

My next thought was familial Hibernian fever, otherwise known as TRAPS (tumor necrosis factor receptor-associated periodic syndrome), which is caused by genetic mutations. These fevers, which can persist for a few days or a few months, occur every six weeks or disappear for years, only to resurface. Testing for this condition had only recently been developed. Eventually, I sent Serge to the new genetic testing facility at another hospital.

The results surprised both of us: it was familial Mediterranean fever after all. The odds of inheriting the disease are about 1 in 500. Serge was delighted to finally have a diagnosis, the more so, of course, because the condition is controllable, if not entirely curable, with colchicine, a drug that dates back at least to the time of the ancient Egyptians. An immune system modulator derived from a flower, the autumn crocus, it is also useful in treating gout and rheumatism. Although Serge still occasionally gets a fever, it does not spike as high or last for as long as it once did. More important, we almost certainly prevented the development of amyloidosis, a known complication of familial Mediterranean fever, which can lead to renal failure.

I was raised in Lachine, just outside Montreal. My father was a housepainter and my mother was a bookbinder. As a child — I actually had forgotten this and had to be reminded of it many years later when it became relevant — I suffered from periodic fevers. At the time, we didn't see them as anything more than childhood illnesses, though I apparently had them more often than others. People were always telling me, "Don't get your feet wet because when you do, you get a fever and a sore throat." At one point, they were going to take my tonsils out.

For years, I also suffered from severe stomach cramps, which we know now is a manifestation of familial Mediterranean fever, but at the time was diagnosed as allergies to dairy products or gluten. So I would change my diet and temporarily get better, but the pains would always return. At times, it was intense I'd be on the floor crying. I'd say, "Just kill me. Get it over with."

I earned a bachelor's degree in economics at the University of Waterloo, and in 1977 immediately went to work for Hewlett-Packard. I was there 20 years, first as a systems engineer, and then in sales development, product management and development and then in sales management. Then they sent me to Hong Kong in market development and marketing manager. I was there 11 years. I travelled about 70 percent of the year, covering Asia.

During that time, I earned an executive M.B.A. I left HP in 1994, at age 40, and started consulting in sales development, based in Hong Kong. I returned to Toronto in 1999 and became involved in various businesses — an accounting firm that I co-owned, a restaurant in which I was a silent partner and a family company in the mining business in Quebec. I still play a marginal role there, but I have largely retired.

In 2005, I became ill, emotionally and physically. I discovered that my partner was committing fraud and had to sue him, creating a lot of stress. Physically, I had abdominal pain and high fevers — 103, 104 degrees — and weight loss. The fevers lasted a few days to several days and every night I'd wake up in a pool of sweat. I had memory issues, sleep issues, joint pains. I was depressed and debilitated. It all impacted me.

It took seven years in total to diagnose the illness. Before then, I had every test possible: MRIs, CT scans, x-rays, lumbar punctures, upper GI scopes, lower GI scopes. Every week almost I was tested for HIV. Everything was negative. I saw rheumatologists, autoimmune specialists, endocrinologists, gastroenterologists, infectious disease doctors.

I was three years with Dr. Mourad and about four with Dr. Ho Ping Kong. We had to wait a long time, almost a year, for genetic testing, first to get provincial approval and then do the sample and send them away to the United States for analysis; we did not have the facilities here.

They ultimately told me FMF is a rare genetic order that affects mainly Semites, about 1 in 200. I apparently have a mutation upon the mutation, a real anomaly. My first thought was "Where the hell did that come from?" And the next was "Well, maybe we can address it now."

It was very odd, because to get FMF you have to inherit genes from both parents. On my father's side, we can trace the family back to Paris in the 17th century. On my mother's side, it's all French Roman Catholic for 100 years. My mother's father came from Manchester but, as far as we know, he was not Jewish and even then I'd need a gene from my father's side.

When I met Dr. Ho Ping Kong, we had immediate rapport, in part because he speaks French, but also because he just puts you at ease. He's a patient-oriented doctor. We could have a conversation. A lot of doctors talk to you as if you'd been to medical school. HPK speaks in words you can understand. It never felt like a medical lecture. It was comforting. He gave me a sense of hope. I intuitively knew: this man knows a lot, though I can't tell you why. He has seen a lot. If there is going to be a solution, he will find it. And he did. I still have occasional fevers, but the drug helps modulate them. I still have stomach cramps but they are also less intense.

NOT EVERY ILLNESS NEEDED TRIALS and studies in order to determine the best therapeutic response. Years of experience with penicillin had demonstrated incontrovertibly that it would cure patients with pneumonia. The same was true for mitral stenosis and atrial fibrillation, a scourge of young people for many years, because of rheumatic fever. In that population, strokes were 25 times more common than in the general population. We did not need elaborate studies to know that the best treatment to prevent strokes in mitral stenosis was anti-coagulation therapy, despite the risks of bleeding.

Until the emergence of people like Sackett and Feinstein, only 15–20 percent of our decision-making was based on hard scientific evidence. The new approach laid a much greater emphasis on the conduct of clinical trials, seeking to prove efficacy by the sheer weight of statistical probability. Today, it is estimated that as much as 40 percent is evidence-based, and that figure continues to rise.

Consider, for example, the use of statin drugs like Crestor or Lipitor for cardiac disease. We have long had evidence that if someone had already suffered a heart attack, a statin regimen could help prevent a second infarction. But what about people with high cholesterol readings or a strong genetic predisposition — yet no specific history of heart disease? In such situations, many cardiologists would prescribe statins, which would usually be effective. But each patient required a separate discussion. There was no clear research evidence to support such an approach.

In the mid-1990s, a group in West Scotland conducted a double-blind study involving almost 7,000 men, age 45–64. One group received a placebo; the second was given the drug pravastatin. The first result was perhaps no surprise. The statin lowered plasma cholesterol levels by 20 percent, and low-density-lipoprotein cholesterol levels by 26 percent, versus no change in the placebo group. The second result was more dramatic: 248 coronary events (non-fatal myocardial infarction or death from coronary heart disease) among the placebo group, compared with 174 in the group taking pravastatin.

At Toronto Western, in the mid-1980s, we set up a curriculum for teaching evidence-based medicine. A former resident of mine who became one of the world's leading bioethicists, Dr. Peter Singer, did most of that work. (Peter appears elsewhere in this book with his own views on the art of medicine.) In turn, Singer teamed up with Allan Detsky, director of general internal medicine at Toronto General Hospital. For five years, they offered twice-a-week seminars in clinical epidemiology and evidence-based medicine that drew standing-room-only crowds of students, teaching how to evaluate patient-oriented research papers.

Several later luminaries emerged from that program, all of them making significant contributions to research. Among them was David Naylor, a former colleague who set up the Institute for Clinical Evaluative Sciences (ICES) at Toronto's Sunnybrook Hospital to do independent, non-profit research on a broad range of health-related issues. Its work, in many fields, has been absolutely world class.

For almost two decades, the groundswell for evidence-based science was so strong that voices arguing for medicine as an art were largely marginalized. Today, there is more interest in what physicians do and how they ought to behave — questions that speak to the artistic side of the equation. There seems to be an understanding that perhaps we have gone too far with the scientific model, especially as we better comprehend the importance of personalized medicine — i.e., targeting disease based on an individual's unique genetic makeup.

The best physicians, in my judgment, are those who know the science backwards and forwards, but also demonstrate the distinct human touch. I don't suggest that all doctors need to have those skills. If you are about to undergo brain surgery, what matters most, surely, is the knowledge and talent of the neurosurgeon, not his or her ability to make small talk.

But most physicians, those who deal with patients on a one-to-one basis, need to have some of these qualities. You may learn some of this sensitivity by studying history and literature before entering medical school, but I think, in general, that you are who you are. You bring your genes and your attitude to the bedside with you. The onus thus falls heavily on boards of admission to choose wisely in selecting applicants.

Evidence-based medicine has been an invaluable boon to doctors. It has taught us a great deal about the diagnosis of heart disease, hypertension, various forms of cancer and other illnesses. And it has helped define the gold standards for treatment of these and many other conditions. But I still maintain that evidence-based medicine cannot provide all answers to all doctors. The profession's Grey Zone is simply too large — too many patients with clinical symptoms, clearly in need of treatment, but no reliable diagnoses. And there are too many questions that the evidence of trials and studies cannot satisfactorily answer. Thus, there will be a continuing need for the art of medicine — the importance of experience, empathy, communication, intuition, and knowing and doing the right thing.

IN 1978, WHILE WORKING AT the Royal Victoria Hospital in Montreal, I was asked to consult on a case involving Andrei, a middle-aged Haitian man said to be suffering from pulmonary tuberculosis. He was one of the cases we discussed during our weekly ward meetings. He had all the signs of TB — fever, cough, weight loss and sweating.

What was particularly curious about his story was that he had been treated for the same disease three months earlier and ostensibly had been cured. Or so it was believed. Now the disease had returned, although its principal symptoms were less active. But in the interim, Andrei had lost his eyesight. The eyes are sometimes affected by TB, but rarely to the point of blindness. So we were all puzzled and struggled with the diagnosis. Nobody asked about sexual orientation. It wasn't remotely on our radar at the time. We treated him for TB a second time, but to no avail. He died soon afterward.

Six months later, another Montreal hospital asked me to examine a 21-year-old patient from Barbados suffering from what they said was Still's disease, an inflammatory arthritic condition. But as soon as I saw him, I knew this was the wrong diagnosis. The poor man was wasting away; he'd lost something like 50 pounds in a mere six months. We looked for evidence of tuberculosis, autoimmune disorders, rheumatoid diseases and infection. But there was nothing specific we could find, and nothing, unfortunately, that we could do. Not long afterwards, he succumbed as well.

It was only in hindsight that it became clear to me that these two cases were among the first, if not the first, cases of HIV/AIDS in Canada. They had occurred several years before this terrible disease began to make its presence felt in North America. I can't definitively prove that these two Montreal patients actually were victims of AIDS — at the time, we did not save serum samples — but I am convinced that they were. Ten years later, the problems Andrei was having with his eyes would have been labelled CMV retinitis, a classic complication of HIV/AIDS.

In the medical literature, the first North American case was reported on June 5, 1981, by the Centers for Disease Control and Prevention citing five incidences of pneumocystis carinii pneumonia (PCP) among previously healthy young gay men in Los Angeles. Two had died.

Soon enough, however, reports began to filter in of young homosexual men dying in significant numbers in major American and Canadian cities. At first, we labeled it "gay bowel syndrome." Patients would initially report severe diarrhea and weight loss. They would deteriorate from there. While the medical community recognized what was happening, many hospitals simply did not want to treat these patients. Our caseload at Toronto Western Hospital typically included young men from small or mid-sized rural communities whose own institutions had effectively turned them away. People were too scared to admit these patients.

Even at Toronto Western Hospital, where the efforts of doctors and nurses were, in my judgment, heroic, we informally capped the number of hospitalized AIDS patients at 20, fearing that we would otherwise compromise other aspects of the care program. We thought other hospitals needed to do their fair share. We incurred criticism for putting that ceiling in place, and we were accused of being homophobic, but it had to be done. But two of my colleagues demonstrated remarkable conviction and grace under pressure — Dr. Doug McFadden, a general internist who led the effort at Western. He had a Ph.D. in epidemiology and an open mind, and he became the first real HIV doctor in Toronto. Our second stalwart was Ann McMahon, a Scottish-born head nurse of exceptional talent, commitment and compassion, a modern incarnation of Florence Nightingale.

At one point, we faced an ethical dilemma, whether to hire a male nurse who had already been diagnosed with the disease. On the one hand, we wanted to do the right thing vis-à-vis human rights and non-discrimination. On the other, we needed to do — and be perceived as doing — the right thing for patients in the face of a growing pandemic. In the end, we decided that hiring the nurse for ward duties would inadvertently expose far more patients to what we believed was substantial risk.

The move provoked something of an uproar in the gay community, and I was cast as the villain. But it was the right decision, especially as we better came to understand the risks posed by transmission of the virus through accidental needle pricks. That happens routinely in hospitals, and it happened at Western; fortunately, no HIV/AIDS cases resulted.

On occasion, patients would turn up from all over the world showing all the symptoms of AIDS but not want us to perform a confirming blood test. Such cases posed a problem for us because, as matter of public health, just as we routinely do for syphilis, we should do the test. But legally, we did not have the right to compel the patient to undergo testing.

But HIV certainly changed the way we look at medicine. Before its emergence, we tended to classify disease illness as infectious, or inflammatory, or cancerous, or congenital or metabolic. HIV could be several of these things at once. It was hard to know where one category ended and the next started, and what to treat first. It was an infection that could lead to cancer and inflammation, with patients presenting with muscle and joint pain, anemia, peripheral neuropathy, blindness, brain disease, encephalitis, not only ordinary pneumonias and tuberculosis, but also more exotic forms to which a compromised immune system was vulnerable — diseases we otherwise rarely saw. It also changed hospital procedures, with barrier protection becoming commonplace.

Debate still rages in the medical community over whether a French or an American team of researchers discovered HIV — human immunodeficiency virus — first. Regardless, the cocktail of anti-viral drugs eventually assembled for treatment has made it more manageable, a chronic as opposed to a universally progressive fatal disease.

THE FRIGHTENING SPEED WITH WHICH epidemics can move had already been brought home to me. In 1975, I was looking after a group of about 40 Canadian war veterans in Montreal. On a certain Friday in the dead of winter, an influenza germ found its way onto the ward. By Monday morning, 28 of my patients were dead. Their elderly immune systems were simply too compromised to fight the disease. That event had a profound influence on my thinking about epidemics.

I had seen epidemics before, of course. In 1964, during my fourth year in medical school in Jamaica, a typhoid fever epidemic struck the country — a staggering 4,000 cases. Typhoid is a tough, highly communicable disease, with a high mortality rate. It has a long duration that begins with fever and constipation and then progresses. By its third week, it infects the lymphoid tissue of the small bowel, resulting in diarrhea. By the fourth week, untreated, you will be near death from toxemia or bleeding.

Enrolled in a course called social and preventative medicine, three other students and I were dispatched to the countryside to help with the investigation. We visited one hospital near the epicentre of the epidemic. In each cot were two kids, lying foot to head, both suffering from typhoid fever. They simply did not have enough beds though, fortunately, they did have sufficient antibiotics.

We visited the origin of the outbreak — a rural river in which the mother of the first typhoid patient had washed his soiled clothes. That was the index case. Three weeks later, a mile downstream, 10 new cases were reported. Then, further downstream, a fortnight later, another 100 cases. The incubation period was 14 days and then it was from person to person. It was a classic, natural history of a waterborne epidemic.

But my formal introduction to epidemiology occurred later, during the 1968 Hong Kong flu epidemic. Only a medical intern at the time, I watched sadly as two young men experienced acute respiratory distress, then heart failure and finally died. Such experiences eventually led countries to develop programs in public health. We realized then that social and preventive medicine would become a major factor in the ongoing struggle to keep people healthy.

THREE DECADES LATER, TORONTO CONFRONTED another pandemic — SARS, severe acute respiratory syndrome. I recall its genesis vividly. It was Sunday, March 16, 2003. I had just returned from a winter holiday. My son, Wayne, a cardiologist at the Scarborough Hospital (Grace campus) — it would become the epicentre of the epidemic — came to visit me and said he needed his children to stay with me. He would not be going home for at least two weeks.

I was initially confused. "What are you saying to me? Are you serious?"

"I am," he said. "There are 100 cases of an undiagnosed disease at the hospital, and people are dying."

An occasional hospital colleague announced that he was taking holidays rather than expose himself to the as-yet-unidentified virus. His cardiology partner had decided to sleep in the family basement, to avoid the risk of spreading the presumed germ to his wife and children. Wayne, and his partners, Dr. Chris Li, Dr. David

Rose, and Dr. Sandy Finkelstein and their hospital colleagues, were to perform heroic work in taking care of the 100 SARS patients at Scarborough Grace.

The next day at Toronto Western Hospital, my team assessed the situation. We were just beginning to understand what was going on, but events were moving quickly. The Centers for Disease Control in Atlanta had just conducted its first briefing, reporting 14 suspected SARS cases under investigation in the U.S. Our staff had to be prepared, both logistically and psychologically, for the possibility that we would be soon admitting SARS patients. That same night, we did — a 60-year-old Chinese gentleman, transferred from the intensive care unit at Mount Sinai Hospital and considered stable. We placed him in a special, isolated room with negative pressure. It turned out that he was the husband of one of the first victims to contract the illness in Hong Kong, not far from Guangdong, China, where the outbreak had begun the previous fall. His wife had likely given him the virus.

When we first prepared to examine him, we were fortunate enough to have a Cantonese-speaking medical student on our team; the patient himself spoke no English. We were lucky, too, to have a courageous and knowledgeable intern who ultimately supervised the case, Dr. Avijit Chatterjee. It was his suggestion — actually, his insistence — that we all be double gowned, double gloved and double masked. Today, that protective ensemble would be routine for epidemic situations, but at the time it was novel.

In fact, I was initially surprised by the recommendation and asked him why we needed to do it.

"Trust me," he said. "I have a master's degree in microbiology from McGill University. This is what we need to do."

Even then, we did not have as much physical contact with the patient as we have under ordinary circumstances, though we did make sure that he was stable and was breathing normally. He survived his ordeal.

In total, we ourselves recorded 29 SARS cases at TWH — about

15 percent of all reported or suspected Canadian cases. Four deaths occurred at Toronto Western Hospital (there were 43 in all of Canada), all in the ICU. But there were no additional infections. One reason why the death total at Western was so low was because we put our SARS patients in rooms with negative pressure, which prevents the spread of potentially fatal germs.

I witnessed several acts of heroism during that traumatic period, but few were more impressive that those of infectious disease specialist Wayne Gold. He examined every one of the SARS patients we admitted. Gold's performance, duplicated by dozens of health care professionals in Ontario — many of them from the younger generation — had an enormous impact. Dr. Gold was the sole attending physician for those patients admitted, which meant we did not have to pass patients from one physician to the next, as occurred at other institutions.

The SARS epidemic fundamentally changed the way Canadians perceived nurses and doctors, reducing complaints about the system dramatically and for several years.

Many mysteries remain from that pandemic, however. Why were some people more susceptible to the germ than others? Why did some live and others die? My son's secretary became ill. Although she survived, she must have passed it on to her father, who did not. One of his own partners in cardiology became ill with SARS and, though he recovered, he decided to take early retirement.

SARS was, of course, a new disease, caused by a new virus for which we had no immunity, no specific antibodies. Although some deaths occurred among young people, most of those who died were elderly, with immune systems already somewhat compromised by other conditions. Among the young, the body's own immune response mechanisms can be part of the problem, kicking into such high gear that, in concert with the virus itself, they overwhelm the ability of organs to function.

It was probably because there were so many unknowns that so many of us found the crisis unnerving. We intended to manage it with fidelity to the best practices of pandemic control. But would those be sufficient to corral the virus? We just didn't know. For the first week or so, I found myself occasionally waking in the middle of the night, bathed in sweat, my heart racing and unable to get back to sleep. I was not alone; I know this anxiety was felt in many medical households. We suffered but we persevered as a profession.

We had some other close calls. One day, at the virtual height of the crisis, I was treating Samantha, a woman with Addison's, a rare disease of the adrenal glands. Her blood pressure had fallen to about 100 and she felt tired and depressed. Her skin colour had also changed, becoming more pigmented, a common feature of the disease — the result of low cortisol levels. We sent her to Toronto General for an ACTH test to confirm the diagnosis.

She had been administered the test and was leaving the hospital when, in the elevator, she collapsed. Respirologist Dr. Michael Hutcheon found her and, tracing her file, called me. Her blood pressure had now fallen to 80, he reported. His question was: should he send her to Toronto General's emergency department or did I want to come and get her?

I had to make an instant decision. The easier option would have been to let her go to emergency. But I had a medical student with me and, thinking this might be a teachable moment for her, told the TGH doctor that we would take the next shuttle bus and bring Samantha back to Toronto Western. At the same time, I called a colleague of mine at Mount Sinai, Dr. Shabbir Alibhai, and asked him to cross the street to Toronto General and check on her first, to make sure she was okay. If he had said she was in bad shape, I'd have been tempted to send her to emergency and I would have met her there.

As it turned out, it was on that day that SARS appeared in TGH's emergency department. Four people there subsequently died and three staff members developed SARS. I sensed disaster looming. Had I sent Samantha there, given her already weakened condition, she would have been extremely vulnerable to the virus. So would have I, or anyone on the ward that day. At best, we would have all been quarantined.

But the key factor was my student. I wanted her to experience something about the art of medicine, specifically about empathy. You always want to act in ways that you think will be best for the patient. In this case, that meant not dispatching her to the strange impersonality of another hospital's emergency ward and to physicians she did not know. She was my patient and therefore my responsibility, with or without the SARS crisis. The right thing to do, if I could, was to take the higher ethical road. Do what you should do and then do more. The right thing to do was to get her. We went and brought her back to my office at Toronto Western. More than a decade later, Samantha is doing very well, her disease under control. And she — and we — likely dodged a serious bullet.

AN

INTERNIST'S

PERSPECTIVE

Dr. DAVID FROST

*Dr. David Frost is a staff general internist at the University Health
Network, and a clinician/teacher at the Centre for Excellence in
Education and Practice at Toronto Western Hospital.*

JUST 32 YEARS OLD, AND only a few years removed from his chief residency in internal medicine, Dr. David Frost is among the youngest of the physicians recruited to work in Dr. Herbert Ho Ping Kong's Centre for Excellence in Education and Practice (CEEP). Although he says he derives most enjoyment from direct patient care, he devotes research time to an issue that looms over the health care system — the disproportionate use of resources (in dollars, equipment and medical personnel) by a very small percentage of the population.

"My work looks at optimizing patients with multi-system medical problems and seeking ways to care for them that reduce hospital readmissions," he explains. Such patients constitute about one percent of the population, but account for 30–40 percent of total expenditures. This lopsided statistic is the result of a paradox. On the one hand, improvements in the broader health care system mean people are living longer. But precisely because they live longer, they are more likely to develop what are known as "co-morbidities," overlapping chronic diseases such as diabetes, congestive heart failure and cancer.

"These patients, a tiny percentage of the population, in the last months of their lives represent a hugely disproportionate drain on health resources," Frost says. "The challenge is to identify who are they before they become high users of the system and keep them treated as outpatients. It's a very complex issue with many stakeholders, but we need to get on top of the problem if we are going to have a sustainable health system."

Frost says his medical ambitions began in childhood. "I don't really understand why — I'm the only one in my family crazy enough to go into medicine — but there was never been a doubt in my mind that that's what I wanted to do, and it was always the only thing I wanted to do. As I grew up, the academic side of medicine appealed to me." Later, in medical school, although he considered anesthesia and surgery, he chose general internal medicine because it offered "direct patient care with an academic side. I was more suited to being a generalist than a specialist. For me, the broader knowledge base was more appealing."

As an acolyte of Dr. Ho Ping Kong, Frost has tried to emulate some of his practices. One of these is making regular visits to the radiology department to talk to the specialists who read MRIs, CT scans and ultrasound images.

"Herbert goes every week with a list of his patients who have had tests because, while he will have already read the formal report, he wants to dig deeper," Frost says. "It's surprising because, when you actually speak to the radiologist, things are often not as certain as they might make it seem in the report. They may have insights they don't actually put into the report or ideas they won't share in writing for medical-legal reasons or because they may appear too speculative."

Frost recalls a case in which the patient presented with fever, weight loss and leg pain. She had developed a hematoma in the leg, which made imaging tests difficult to read. "It was very difficult to sort out whether we were seeing blood leaking into the muscle or an underlying mass. The radiologists and people who deal with soft tissue tumours did not know. Herbert was concerned about cancer and advised taking a biopsy, even though we had been told it was not possible and might make things worse. We never were able to override those objections. Months later, we did the biopsy and confirmed a carcinoma. The patient eventually died. But Herbert was helpful in making me question conventional thinking."

Frost says the exponential explosion of medical information makes it increasingly hard for general practitioners to play the role of quarterback in the affairs of patients with multi-system disease. "I think GPs — and my own wife is one of them — do an excellent job overall. They have a very difficult job, perhaps the most difficult in the health care system, staying up-to-date on every aspect of medicine, particularly given the volume of patients. But for certain patient populations, it's just not feasible for a GP to address all the issues in a 10-minute appointment. We need to do a better job of supporting them, and I think that will lead to a growing role for the general internist."

Complicating the situation is the system of subspecialization, which he says is necessary in treating many conditions, but "does have consequences." Subspecialists may not have a full awareness of other ailments the patient is dealing with, or they may offer advice that directly conflicts with suggestions made by another subspecialist treating a separate disease.

At Toronto Western Hospital, Frost runs a clinic in family practice, in which he liaises regularly with GPs. "That model could be more widespread and could use electronic records to identify patients with multi-system disease," he suggests. "That might be a way to directly provide support to family physicians. It's definitely on the radar of policy thinkers."

Over the past five decades, Frost says, technology has dramatically changed the way medicine is practised. But if technology's role is no longer up for debate, it should not lead, he adds, to an abandonment of traditional ways of coming to a diagnosis. In fact, the physical exam, which most patients expect, can be used to determine the extent of further testing required.

"You don't need to do an echocardiogram on every patient," he says. "But you need to know enough about benign and less benign heart murmurs to know when to order that test. The art of medicine here is using resources wisely. Having the technology makes it easier on the one hand to pick up these murmurs, but harder because you have to interpret them, know when to order them and, increasingly, to justify doing so."

Frost acknowledges the importance of the physical exam and says that in some cases "it is more reliable than the expensive test." Still, he thinks it is less important than it was 30 years ago, "because the same information can be gleaned in other ways, albeit at great expense. Some of the minutiae of ways of coming to diagnosis might be academically interesting, but they don't make a huge difference to actual patient care today."

The aspect of the art of medicine that needs more attention, he says, is ongoing patient care — managing what may be inflated expectations of a physician's ability to diagnose and cure and conveying bad news. "There are guidelines, but they are very hard to standardize. Do you touch the patient? Should you sit or stand? What is the right tone of voice? What is the proper setting? I think you learn this from observing people who are good at it."

The other major challenge, Frost allows, is time. Physicians are under constant pressure to "move cases along, keep lengths of in-patient stay short, come up with disposition plans, make management decisions quickly. It's a challenge to balance all of that with the need to take the extra time needed to establish rapport with the patient. But taking the time to ask where someone is from, or what kind of work they do, can go a long way to putting them at ease and getting important information from them."

CHAPTER 11

CONFRONTING
RARE DISEASES

Medicine is a science of uncertainty and an art of probability.
— Sir William Osler

ONE OF THE MOST CHALLENGING aspects of a career in diagnostic internal medicine is the opportunity it inevitably presents to treat rare diseases. Typically, patients arrive in our offices after a primary health care physician and two or more specialists have done as much as they can and then, metaphorically, thrown up their hands and asked for diagnostic help.

Sometimes, the right answer turns out to have been hiding in plain sight. But just as often, the solution is difficult because it involves a rare, seldom-seen disease. Both the diagnostic process and the subsequent treatment are important aspects of the art of medicine.

Some years ago, I was invited to become consulting physician in internal medicine to a professional sports team in Toronto. The players needed attention from various specialists, including of course orthopedic surgeons, but they very seldom felt the need to seek my services. They were essentially too healthy. Then someone suggested it might be more useful if I consulted on members of the team's executive management, so I agreed.

Thus did I get to meet John C., then 62 years old. Although initially reluctant, he did allow me to take a family history. Among other things, it indicated a genetic predisposition for colonic polyps, and I eventually persuaded him to have a colonoscopy. As it turned out, he had more than 100 polyps, which are generally considered precursors for colon cancer. Needless to say, he was very grateful. After the polyps were removed, we worked on a new regimen for diet, exercise and blood pressure control.

Some months later, I bumped into John in the hospital atrium and immediately noticed he was limping and dragging his leg.

"What's the matter?"

"I'm not sure," he said. "This happened last night. I just feel a little funny."

"Well, go upstairs. It's important to examine you."

It did not take long to discover that he had a hemiparesis, a partial paralysis, affecting an entire side of his body. It was the result, I suspected, of a small stroke. An MRI later confirmed that diagnosis. It had affected an important part of the brain but, fortunately, only a small portion.

I gave John another lecture at that point on the importance of diet, exercise and staying on his medications.

John travelled frequently to the United States with his pro team. On one of his next trips, he fell into conversation with a rival executive who denigrated the quality of medical care John was receiving in Canada. He advised him to come to the U.S. where, he assured him, surgeons could perform angioplasty — essentially, a balloon opening — for the blood vessel in his brain.

When John returned, he conferred with me and others about that idea. After sending him to see a Toronto neurologist, we recommended a conservative approach that, for the moment, excluded angioplasty. We had made the assumption that there was some atherosclerosis in the brain, but we considered surgery too dangerous at that point.

"The choice is yours," I explained to him, "but we think it's more prudent to be less aggressive."

He agreed. "If you say, 'Don't do it,' I won't do it."

John did well for the next few years. He made a full recovery from the stroke, regaining his strength and his ability to walk without a limp. But one day, he suffered a cardiac arrest while sitting at his desk. He might have died, except that a colleague happened to pass by his office within two minutes of the event and saw him slumped over. He immediately called 911 and began to administer cardiac massage. John was very lucky. The survival rate for heart attack victims that suffer unwitnessed cardiac arrests is very low.

Interestingly, a subsequent angiogram indicated there were no serious blockages in his coronary arteries. In other words, he did not have conventional coronary artery disease.

Again, John made a good recovery and returned to work. Two years later while attending a social function, he experienced acute abdominal pain and was rushed to an emergency ward. I saw him the next day and ordered a CT scan that revealed swelling of the bowel. An astute colleague, imaging specialist Anthony Hanbidge, suggested it might be amyloidosis, a rare, not well-understood disease. In my lifetime, I have seen it less than half a dozen times.

In fact, it is safe to say there is more that we don't yet know about the pathophysiology of amyloidosis than we do. What we know is that it creates amyloids, deposits of fibrous proteins, which interfere with the normal functioning of the body. We also know that it has been implicated in a wide variety of diseases, including Alzheimer's, diabetes, Parkinson's and heart arrhythmias — the very kind that might have precipitated John's cardiac arrest. Moreover, amyloidosis is related to multiple myeloma, a cancer of the white blood cells.

If Hanbidge's assessment was correct, we should have been

able to find distinct markers for amyloid in the blood, including so-called immunoglobulin light chains — defective proteins involved in the body's immune system. There's another indicia for the disease — dark, purplish rings around the eyelids; John, it turned out, had these, too. We biopsied the eyelid tissue and confirmed the presence of amyloids. Finally, we did a bone marrow test and it, too, confirmed the diagnosis.

So a mystery had finally been solved. John's ailments through the years — the stroke, the cardiac arrest and the bowel disorder — were in the end the result of a single rare disease, amyloidosis. It is potentially lethal, but also potentially treatable. John was given chemotherapy and responded well.

The art of medicine often involves precisely this kind of difficult process, where the clinician struggles to identify the interrelationship of symptoms and to integrate knowledge that may affect different organs over a long period of time. But you have to follow the clues. A cardiac arrest that was not caused by arterial blockages should have alerted us to the possibility of amyloidosis earlier.

In a similar case, I was recently introduced to Gregory, a 64-year-old university professor. He'd been an athlete in his youth and had remained active, carefully watching his diet and his weight. After experiencing some shortness of breath, he'd been to another hospital and been diagnosed with hypertrophic cardiomyopathy, a genetic disease in which the muscles of the heart harden or thicken. If the muscles enlarge in the wrong places, they can interfere with the organ's delicate balance of rhythm and cause sudden death. Athletes often have enlarged hearts and are thus more susceptible to complications in the organ.

Despite the diagnosis, confirmed by listening to the heart and an MRI, Gregory was insistent that something else was going on. He had complained to his family doctor of feeling tiredness in his legs when he walked. He could only complete half his usual routine on a treadmill.

At that point, he was referred to me. More than most patients, he was assertive in pushing for tests that would get to the bottom of things.

"Well, there is a heart problem, because we can hear it," I told him. "And the weariness in your legs may be a natural consequence of what's happening in the heart. Your heart isn't pumping as well as it should."

"Absolutely not," he insisted. "The legs are a separate issue."

I then suggested we take another, closer look at the heart. In fact, Toronto General Hospital runs a clinic especially for patients with hypertrophic cardiomyopathy. I wanted to send him there.

"Don't send me there," he pleaded. "I was warned that they would do invasive procedures and then start chopping up my heart."

Apart from the heart, his physical exam was normal, except for some mild parasthesia — tingling — in his feet.

"If I'm right," he said, "and it's not just the heart, what could it be?"

"It could be spinal stenosis," I said. "At your age, you're entitled to have some arthritis. That may affect bony parts of your spine, which impinge on the spinal cord and give you these feelings of tiredness when you walk. We call it spinal claudication."

A good theory, perhaps, but erroneous. A subsequent MRI showed no compression of the spine.

My next idea was to consult with a colleague, cardiologist Dr. John Janevski. After reviewing the case, he noted that Gregory's heart voltage readings were lower than they should have been — a potentially important clue. The best option, we agreed, was to send him to the hypertrophic cardiomyopathy clinic — the very place he was refusing to go.

We continued to do battle — Gregory maintaining that his heart was not the cause of his leg fatigue and me insisting that it was. Somehow, Dr. Janevski and I managed to persuade him to visit the clinic and see Dr. Harry Rakowski, among the world's reigning experts on the condition. It did not take long for Rakowski to report back, but the diagnosis surprised all of us — cardiac amyloidosis. A bone marrow test later confirmed the presence of amyloid, protein-rich deposits that gradually replace heart muscle and impair the organ's function. The patient promptly began chemotherapy but, sadly, it was by then too late. He succumbed soon afterward.

MANY RARE DISEASES, OF COURSE, are rare only in the context of the developed world. In my native Jamaica and in the tropical Third World generally, the rare can be quite common. Perhaps with my origins in mind, a colleague once sent me a patient that he suspected was suffering from a disease known as ciguatera. Well known in the Caribbean, it is caused by toxins that may reside within several varieties of reef fish. Eating the fish can give you the disease. It also gave me one of the most complex cases I have ever dealt with.

Nigel was a retired businessman of about 70. He had a history of coronary heart disease and had received a triple bypass some years previously. It did not relate directly to the reported diagnosis of ciguatera, but it was something to consider in terms of possible drug treatments.

After the initial episode of vomiting and diarrhea in the Bahamas, Nigel returned home and soon started to complain of chronic fatigue, with acute pain and tingling of the hands and feet. The pain was severe enough to interrupt his sleep. Eventually, these symptoms subsided, but then returned, with swelling in his legs. His family doctor thought it might be polymyalgia rheumatica, an autoimmune disorder, and prescribed prednisone. If it was PMR, then the drug would likely alleviate his symptoms. In fact, after the first day, he was much better. But on the second day, he relapsed and by the third day was so sick that he stopped the medication.

His GP then sent him to Dr. Jay Keystone, an infectious disease specialist. He thought Nigel's symptoms might have been the legacy of his encounter with ciguatera, but recommended I see him. I confessed to no special expertise, despite my Caribbean background, but found a resident eager to explore the ciguatera mystery. Little did we know how difficult and complex Nigel's case would become.

A series of blood tests quickly revealed inflammation of some kind — above normal levels of ESR and C-reactive protein. Those results supported the family doctor's diagnosis — polymyalgia rheumatica (PMR). In the meantime, my colleague Dr. David Frost examined Nigel and discovered that his fingers were over-sized and spade-like. It was Frost who first raised the possibility of acromegaly, a rare disease caused by excess production of the human growth hormone in the brain's pituitary gland. Spade-like fingers is one sign of the disease.

Interestingly, it takes seven years on average to make an acromegaly diagnosis — precisely the length of time Nigel had complained of his symptoms — because its manifestations unveil themselves so slowly. And the disease typically affects middle-aged men. Rare though it is, acromegaly has affected many famous people including U.S. president Abraham Lincoln, motivational speaker Tony Robbins and former heavyweight champion boxer Primo Carnera.

Frost's diagnosis remained, for the moment, speculative, though it was supported by other evidence as well, including carpal tunnel syndrome. If you shook Nigel's hand, he literally screamed in pain. The pain was so intense that he had become deeply depressed; we enlisted a psychiatrist to try and help. We prescribed an anti-depressant medication to help him sleep, but he continued to lament his condition and insist there was no point in living like this.

We ordered yet another CT scan, this time concentrating on his frontal lobe. It revealed enlarged sinuses, yet another feature of acromegaly. Sensing that we were closer to a firm diagnosis, we reexamined his hands. They showed changes of the terminal phalanx, the bones at the tips of our fingers, also compatible with the ailment.

Finally, we x-rayed his feet and compared the results against an x-ray taken three years earlier. It showed that his heel pad had grown from 21 to 26 millimetres. By then, we were beginning to feel confident we had found the right answer — a long way from the original diagnosis, ciguatera. Acromegaly is usually amenable to hormonal treatment and, if necessary, surgery to remove the pituitary tumour that causes it.

On his next visit, I told Nigel that I doubted whether ciguatera was the cause of his problems. The changes in sensation in his hands suggested peripheral neuropathy — some degree of nerve entrapment at the wrist, caused by carpal tunnel syndrome. We sent him to see Dr. Robert Chen, a specialist in nerve conduction, who confirmed median nerve neuropathy — in other words, carpal tunnel syndrome (CTS).

Despite that finding, Dr. Chen wasn't convinced that it was CTS alone; he thought it could be vasculitis, a rare (1 in 2,000) autoimmune condition in which the body essentially attacks its own blood vessels. The same thought had already occurred to me, and I had ordered a CT angiogram scan to test for what is known as medium vessel vasculitis. It proved negative.

Nigel, meanwhile, continued to suffer. He reported severe pain in his arms, knees and hands, which continued to swell. I knew that relatively minor surgery on the hands could relieve the pain, so that was scheduled and performed. But while the swelling was reduced, he insisted that he was not appreciably better. However, nerve conduction tests conducted four weeks showed marked improvement and validated the carpal tunnel diagnosis.

My own instinct, though it seemed impossible to prove, was

that his family doctor's instinct had been correct — this was likely polymyalgia rheumatica. PMR is another one of those Grey Zone diseases that can never be definitively proven or disproven. But his range of symptoms was most consistent with that condition.

Then Nigel himself, who had a doctor in the family, came up with his own suggestion — a milder variant of PMR known as RS3PE. Its real name is remitting seronegative symmetrical synovitis with pitting edema, which makes its abbreviation to alpha-numeric form entirely understandable.

Nigel's did indeed exhibit several symptoms characteristic of RS3PE, including carpal tunnel syndrome and swelling of his hands. But by any name, the treatment would be the same — prednisone, on a reducing dosage, over a year to 18 months, starting at 20 milligrams. Given his prior adverse reaction, Nigel was reluctant to start the therapy. But he eventually agreed, and within days, he sent me an email reporting that he was much improved and having fun. PMR tends to be an illness that burns itself out after a period of time. Hopefully, that will be Nigel's experience as well.

A PATIENT'S PERSPECTIVE — *Nigel E.* ————————

About six years ago, I was stricken with ciguatera, a fish toxin in the Bahamas. It looks like food poisoning, but isn't. It comes on really fast and violently. People can die of dehydration very quickly. It's like lead poisoning and then starts to destroy your peripheral nerves, and thus starts to look like diabetes. I was very tired and kept going to my doctor and walked around with this for years. I had all kinds of tests. Dr. Keystone wasn't sure what to do and sent me to see Dr. Ho Ping Kong. I've changed his name, by the way. It's not Dr. Ho Ping to Find A Cure. It's Dr. Will Find A Cure.

Now, we're having a debate. He think it's PMR and I think it's RS3PE. One of the differences is bilateral systemic swelling in the hands. They took some readings of the nerve that showed poor conduction, so they did surgery to relieve the nerve. And the nerve problem is common in RS3PE, but abnormal in polymyalgia rheumatica. Then there's dorsal pitting of hands and feet, which I had. I also had a meniscus problem in my knee, which I had surgically repaired, but the swelling and inflammation came back. And that, too, is characteristic of RS3PE. I'm 70 years old now, so this is what I do. My son, a pediatrician, told me about the disease and I researched it. What difference does the diagnosis make? With RS3PE, you are on the same drug, prednisone, but at a lower dose. So I'm pushing for my diagnosis so I can take a lower dose and hopefully have fewer side effects. I'm also on diabetes drugs. They claim I have diabetes, but I think it's all part of the same syndrome. Prednisone stops the pain. Other medications they tried did not, possibly because those other drugs stop nerve pain and my pain isn't nerve pain. What I like about HPK, among other things, is that you see him every week, and not for 15 minutes. He stays as long as it takes.

THE PRACTICE OF MEDICINE IS a humbling craft. Questions present themselves by the dozens; answers are often illusive. When I was a student, we were convinced that the study of human immunology would soon yield a treasure trove of solutions to a variety of disease puzzles. Immunology remains an exciting field of study, and we have made enormous strides. But our youthful optimism about causes and cures has not been redeemed.

Similarly, in genetics, we believed that if we could only determine the genetic basis of a pernicious disease such as cystic fibrosis (CF), we would be well launched on the road to a cure. In fact, researchers successfully identified the CF gene more than 20 years ago but, while we can now provide much better ancillary care to CF patients, we have produced no magic bullet to replace or repair the defective gene.

I was reminded of just how complicated medicine can be when I met Elizabeth G. She'd been sent to me with two potentially serious conditions. The first was Cushing's syndrome, first described by the brilliant American neurosurgeon Harvey Cushing in the 1930s. (Serving in the U.S. medical corps during the First World War, Cushing was called upon to treat Lieutenant Edward Osler, son of the legendary Sir William Osler, who had been wounded during the battle of Ypres. Alas, he could not be saved.)

Elizabeth had all of its classic symptoms — weight gain, a moon-like face and ulcerative sores in her mouth. The best evidentiary test for the syndrome is urinary free cortisol, and Elizabeth registered a level that was almost off the charts. It turned out her mouthwash contained steroids, which her body had absorbed. The second condition was pemphigus vulgaris, which can be lethal, especially if the sores become infected. It's one of the few genuine emergencies in dermatology. But we were able to treat it successfully with medication.

Then, a new complication materialized — polymyalgia rheumatica (PMR), another autoimmune disorder. PMR manifested for Elizabeth, as it often does, with morning achiness and stiffness in the neck, shoulders and trunk. There was also evidence of inflammation in key blood tests. But like many similar conditions, PMR is a disease that is almost impossible to prove or disprove. There is no specific test. However, if the standard treatment — prednisone — is effective, there's a good chance PMR is to blame.

With pemphigus vulgaris or PMR, the names, in a sense, are somewhat arbitrary since all are very likely offshoots of the same fundamental disorder, faulty immune system mechanisms, and one manifestation can easily morph into something else.

In Elizabeth's case, a diminishing dosage of prednisone over about a year effectively eliminated the worst symptoms of PMR. But we continue to monitor her and regularly check her inflammation levels.

A PATIENT'S PERSPECTIVE — *Elizabeth G.*

One morning in 2008, I woke up with ulcerative sores in my mouth. When they did not go away, I went to my dentist. He conducted an oral exam and ultimately concluded the problem was beyond his ability to solve. He sent me to a periodontist, who examined me and concluded the same thing — out of her league. Then I saw an oral surgeon. Same result. Then I was referred to an oral pathologist at a suburban Toronto hospital. By this time, I'd had three biopsies in search of cancer. All were negative. I'd also tried antibiotics, without effect. She referred me to yet another oral pathologist at Mount Sinai, who did an ultraviolet blood test. That came back positive for something called pemphigus vulgaris, a rare autoimmune disorder. It was very painful.

Then I was referred to Toronto Western Hospital to see Dr. Sanjay Siddha, a dermatologist. In the meantime, however, I'd been put on an antibiotic mouthwash that contained a steroid. I had an adverse reaction, swelling up. I became moon-faced. Later, this was diagnosed as Cushing's syndrome, a complication of the cortisol in the mouthwash. But I did not know it initially. It was at that point that Dr. Siddha sent me to Dr. Ho Ping Kong, because Cushing's isn't a condition he treats. HPK ordered a battery of new tests, MRI, CT scan, an endocrine test, looking for tumours of the adrenal gland. So I was driving in from Oakville every week to see either Siddha or HPK or Dr. Rowena Ridout, the endocrinologist.

I didn't mind because, despite the traffic, it was one-stop shopping. I'd see everyone at the same time. I'd be there the whole day. Fortunately, I had flexibility, because I worked in my husband's office. Prior to being diagnosed, I was in Oakville or Burlington or Mississauga. Weeks would go by, in between appointments, and I was getting no answers. Here, it's all under one roof. It saved me a lot of time.

I continued to work, but had to deal with self-esteem issues because I put on about 40 pounds with the swelling, most of it on my upper trunk. I also developed a hump [lump] on the back of my neck. We did not know what it was at first, but HPK kept saying, "It's a puzzle. We go through a process of elimination and rule out and rule out." Finally, we identified it as the steroid in the mouthwash. I was allergic and ballooned up. The pemphigus can flare at any time. It isn't genetic.

I had a whole regime of different types of medicine, three or four for different periods of time. One of them had side effects for lymphoma, so they watched me closely and had blood work done every month. Management of the illness became my life. I became depressed — that's a big part of it. You get down on yourself, at least until the diagnosis. And even though I was reacting to the steroids, I needed to keep taking them, to reduce the inflammation. I've been on a reducing dosage over two years. It's taken that long to get it under control. But we experimented with different drugs to see what would work and give the least side effects.

Then, just when this seemed to be under control, I woke up one morning with very stiff shoulders. I could not lift my arms. I couldn't move my neck. I couldn't roll over in bed. I thought it was the air conditioning. I went to see my GP, and she thought it might be arthritis. Then I saw another specialist who ruled that out, and suggested I come back to

Western to have it investigated. It turned out to be polymy-algia rheumatica, PMR, another autoimmune disorder.

So I saw HPK, and we started all over again. I was here every week. I couldn't lift the blow-dryer to dry my hair. I needed an Advil to get out of bed, literally. So now this is another autoimmune disorder. I had to take prednisone again and started swelling up again. But I had to take it. I joined Weight Watchers eventually and, weaned off the prednisone, started to lose weight, about 30 pounds. The good news with PMR is that once it's over, you usually don't get it again, though I do get occasional symptoms. But that's my new normal — about 85 percent of what I was. That's how I feel. The mouth, however, is fine. I'm pain free and back to a normal diet. I function. I'm even about to try curling. It takes sometimes more than two hours to get here, but it's worth it. Things happen more quickly and I can see all the specialists, sometimes in team conferences. I trust HPK. He's been amazing with me. He's like a friend, very personable. He always asks about my family. We discuss our cottages. That's why I continue to come. I would not get this treatment anywhere else. I keep my fingers crossed that I won't get another autoimmune problem.

I BELIEVE STRONGLY IN CONSULTATION. I go out of my way to solicit the opinions of other physicians, junior or senior. However much you think you may know, however convinced you may be of your own diagnosis, there will always be someone who knows a little more or comes at the problem from a fresh and instructive perspective.

I was reminded of this lesson not long ago by Henry, a 55-year-old lawyer. He was referred to me after running a virtual marathon of the local medical system. He was plainly suffering from some sort of multi-system disease. One kidney had already been damaged irreparably, and the second had had to be surgically stented to save it.

In addition, he had iritis (painful inflammation of the eye), urticaria (hives), chronic pleuritis (inflammation of the lining of the lungs), pericardial disease (inflammation of the heart membrane) and polyarthritis (inflammation of several bodily joints). In pursuit of an answer to his many problems, he'd seen family doctors, eye specialists, dermatologists, nephrologists, rheumatologists and a cardiologist. When I saw him, he was completely fatigued and his joint inflammation was so severe that he could barely walk.

We quickly came to the obvious conclusion that this was a systemic illness, likely caused by an autoimmune disorder. One of my very bright fourth-year residents suggested it might be lupus — technically known as systemic lupus erythematosus. Although it is more common in women than in men, lupus affects the entire body in precisely the ways it had affected Henry. Predictably, his blood work showed evidence of suppressed hemoglobin and elevated levels of erythrocyte sedimentation and C-reactive protein, both indicia of inflammation. The lab tests also revealed high levels of immunoglobulin M, which would ultimately prove to be the key to the mystery.

I went into my consultative mode and called my Toronto Western Hospital colleague, Dr. Sanjay Siddha, a dermatologist. I explained Henry's myriad symptoms and said we had concluded that he likely had lupus. I wanted Dr. Siddha to perform a biopsy to help us confirm that diagnosis.

He soon did but, even before the results were ready, Dr. Siddha came to see me.

"I know what it is," he said. "It's Schnitzler syndrome."

I had never heard of the ailment.

Then he took out his smartphone and began reading. "Schnitzler syndrome, also known as IgM disease, a rare, autoimmune disorder characterized by chronic hives, bone and joint pain, joint inflammation, fatigue, swollen lymph glands and enlarged spleen and liver. Blood tests show a high concentration of specific gamma globulins of the IgM type. Fewer than 100 cases worldwide have been reported before 2008."

First described by the French dermatologist Liliane Schnitzler in the early 1970s, the disease seems to respond best to the drug anakinra (Kineret). We immediately started Henry on this medication. His response to the drug has been most encouraging. We are continuing to monitor his progress closely.

IN PRACTICE, I PROBABLY SEE more of these rare and exotic illnesses than most physicians. Patients often come to me when other medical consultations have failed to provide an answer. They are difficult to diagnose, and sometimes challenging to treat. But the cases have allowed me to expose students and residents to a broader palette of disease that may help in the years ahead. And in exploring medical mysteries, they demonstrate the critical importance of integrating every aspect of the process — family and personal history, the physical examination — and of learning how to weigh the evidence and make connections that can yield solutions.

CHAPTER 12

EPILOGUE

The value of experience is not in seeing much,
but in seeing wisely.
— Sir William Osler

WHAT DOES IT MEAN TO BE A DOCTOR? There are dozens of valid responses but, for me, fundamentally, to be a doctor is to be the beneficiary of a sacred trust. Your patient entrusts you with his or her most valuable possession — life itself.

It is not an easy matter to win that trust. It must be earned.

Nor is it always easy for the patient to confer it.

For many years, my wife and I have made a practice of spending most of our weekend evenings gliding across the floors of various Toronto dance halls. These are clubs of the old school, with old-school dances — waltzes, rhumbas, cha-chas, etc. It is one of our preferred forms of exercise. Among the regulars I have befriended is Ted H. who acts as the evening's disc jockey. In daily life, Ted is a building contractor. Relatively short in stature, he is strong and self-reliant and, I always surmised, physically fit. About 10 years ago, he had experienced periodic bouts of chest pain (angina), accompanied by dizziness and fatigue. But he never went to doctors, never took pills and never complained about feeling unwell, even to his wife and children.

Once, playing recreational hockey, he separated his shoulder, but continued playing. Finding it dislocated the next morning, he propped himself against a door and forced it back into place.

Then, a few years ago, the heart symptoms became so severe that Ted felt compelled, finally, to mention it to his wife. One Saturday night at the dance hall, she approached me to explain the situation. I was, she insisted, the only doctor he would agree to see.

I examined him the following Monday and immediately sent him for a stress test and a meeting with my cardiology colleague Dr. John Janevski. That led to an angiogram, which revealed two serious arterial blockages. Two weeks later, Ted underwent triple bypass surgery, as well as a procedure to repair an aortic aneurism. His life was saved because I had managed through the years to earn his trust. And I had won it not by practising medicine per se, or by behaving like a doctor, but by living a normal life.

SOME YEARS AGO, I WAS privileged to teach a very bright young medical student named Michael Wong. Originally from Quebec City, he went on to enjoy a distinguished career in oncology, first in Buffalo and now in Los Angeles, where he is also a professor of medicine at the University of Southern California. While at Buffalo's Roswell Park Cancer Institute, he wrote an article comparing how clinicians make decisions to writer Malcolm Gladwell's "blink" moment — "making a correct judgment without quite knowing how they reached it." The ability to perceive patterns and extract significant information "from a thin slice of reality . . . plays an intangible yet crucial role in the practice of medicine and in training young physicians." Wong then described a case from his days as a medical resident.

At one point, we were trying to diagnose an elderly lady who'd been found unconscious in her rooming house. All the interns and residents in our department were stumped. Dr. Ho Ping Kong came in, did a brief physical exam and suggested an ultrasound test for abdominal carcinomatosis. We did the test and a subsequent biopsy found that his diagnosis was correct. When I asked, "How did you do that?" he replied, "I've seen it before, and I learned how it looks." Although difficult to put into words, experienced physicians grasp the subtleties of the way certain illnesses present and can sense when something is amiss.

I have experienced many such "blink" moments during my career, some of them outlined earlier in this book. But, in fact, they are the exception, not the rule. Most diagnoses are made by the careful collection and analysis of all the relevant facts. Indeed, even the "blink" moments, as Michael Wong suggests, are simply a distillation of efforts previously expended and experience acquired.

THE ART OF MEDICINE IS NOT — and cannot be — practised in a vacuum. Whatever success I may have enjoyed as a general internist in Jamaica, London, Edinburgh, Montreal and Toronto has been the result of working within a community of remarkable colleagues, willing to share their time, wisdom and expertise. The insights of surgeons, radiologists, pathologists and many other specialists have been indispensable. I make a point not only of meeting them, but of staying in contact, not only for the sake of collegiality, but because you never know when you might need to seek their advice and counsel. I have called upon them frequently. I owe an enormous debt to them all. It's been a privilege to work in a hospital setting where the quality of clinical work is so high.

I could cite dozens of cases where their knowledge and

observations were vital to making the correct diagnosis. One such case involved Nancy, a 50-year-old woman in apparently perfect health. Her only complaint was that every few months she would experience a bout of vomiting; she came to see me looking for the cause. My routine investigations were all negative, so I sent her to a gastroenterologist, who arranged a CT scan and performed a gastroscopy. Again, everything appeared normal. So we were left without an explanation.

I sent her home and advised her to call me if the vomiting resumed. Several weeks later, it did, on a Friday afternoon. By the time she arrived in my office later that day, the vomiting had stopped and she again seemed normal. But on the chance that it might resume, I suggested she be formally admitted to hospital. My thinking was that it might be advantageous to conduct further investigations while she was experiencing the problem. Sometime later, I received a call from the intern on her ward.

"We'd like to order the ultrasound you requested, Dr. Ho Ping Kong, but if I call radiology at this hour, they are likely to say no, whereas if you make the call . . ."

"Leave it to me," I said.

I then called my colleague, Dr. Anthony Hanbidge, in radiology, and explained the situation.

"Better to do another CT scan," he suggested. "It will show more than the ultrasound."

Soon after, he had the images and on them detected a small, cancerous-appearing lesion, the shape of an apple core, in the small bowel. This kind of lymphoma is one of the most difficult diagnoses to make. Why had the first CT scan missed it? Because it had been looking for pancreatic disease and the small bowel had not been adequately scanned.

We immediately sent Nancy to Dr. Todd Penner, one of our most gifted surgeons. He excised the lesion and she commenced a course of radiation and chemotherapy. She survived some years before the cancer returned and took her life.

So while I have argued that the CT scanner, the MRI and other mechanistic marvels should never serve as the crux of the doctor-patient relationship, cases such as Nancy's demonstrate that modern medicine would be greatly diminished — and outcomes adversely affected — without access to this important technology. It's an invaluable tool kit, for diagnosis, prognosis and follow-up care.

The challenge, of course, is to learn to become wise users of that technology — not to invoke it casually or indiscriminately or excessively. That caution applies for two compelling reasons: first, to avoid adding to the existing burden of rising health care costs; second because, as one of my colleagues observes elsewhere in this book, if we look hard and long enough at virtually any patient, we are almost certain to find something that, on an x-ray or ultrasound or magnetic resonance image, looks worthy of further investigation. In such instances, what you discover will be either innocuous and/or irrelevant to your principal line of inquiry and is apt to throw you off the trail.

The successful practitioner should therefore rely on technology largely to confirm diagnostic judgments already made — made, in most cases, by synthesizing the basic, bedside arts of seeing, listening and palpating, by taking a full history and by conducting a thorough physical examination. This combination, I submit, is most likely to yield the most desirable outcomes.

Let me give you a good example.

Through the years, I have treated many patients with complex medical histories. But few cases were as multi-faceted as that of Phirun, a 62-year-old Cambodian-Canadian I examined recently. He had been ill for many years but, through the tender ministrations of his good wife, who had been a midwife in Cambodia, and modern medical technology, he had managed to stay alive.

Phirun's health problems had begun some two decades earlier when he contracted hepatitis C. He recovered, but not, as we shall see, without causing permanent damage to his liver. About

10 years later, a cyst was spotted above his brain's pituitary gland — what we call a craniopharyngioma, a rare occurrence. Although it was not malignant, the neoplasm can, untreated, impair brain and pituitary function. He underwent surgery to remove as much of it as could be removed and was able to resume a normal life.

Then, when his liver began to show signs of failing further, doctors diagnosed hepatocellular carcinoma. This cancer, unfortunately, is usually an unavoidable death sentence because, by the time it is detected, the cancer has advanced too far to be cured. But after careful assessment, Phirun was deemed a viable candidate for a liver transplant.

In due course, the surgery was successfully performed by an accomplished transplant team at Toronto General Hospital. But his travails were not over. Only a year later, an x-ray turned up evidence of a mass on his lung. It turned out to be metastatic lung cancer, from the primary liver cancer. Again, the leading edge of modern medical technology was brought to bear to save Phirun — video-assisted thoracic surgery (VATS) to remove the cancerous lung mass, performed by a team led by the University Health Network's Dr. Thomas Waddell. It was, Waddell later said, one of the first times he had been able to resect such a metastatic tumour using VATS. And again, Phirun responded well.

Some months later, I received a call from Dr. Waddell. The patient, he explained, was suffering from an unidentified condition — pain, stiffness, fatigue, fever — that, in his judgment, was unconnected to the lung surgery. Phirun had been ailing for at least six months. His liver doctor, Les Lilly, was happy with the transplant. Nurse practitioners tending to Phirun also believed something else was at work. Would I agree to see him?

I was initially reluctant, believing that the diagnostic answer was almost certainly connected to one of his previous conditions. Possibly, it was a reaction to the liver transplant graft. Perhaps it was related to the drugs he was taking to prevent rejection of the new organ. Maybe the liver cancer had spread to another site as hepatocellular cancers are prone to do. What would I be able to add?

"There's definitely something wrong," Waddell said, "but we don't think it's related either to the liver or the lungs."

So I finally agreed. The wear and tear on Phirun from his various ordeals was readily apparent. His eyes were sunken. He could barely walk. And, when I examined him, he was physically depleted, able to generate only a minimal level of muscle strength. The blood work showed evidence of inflammation or systemic illness — his sedimentation rate was 130 (about 10 times normal), although this might well have been caused by some underlying condition. His hemoglobin was low (100). After two visits and weighing all the evidence, I still felt the problem would be a legacy of his other illnesses.

On the other hand, two senior and highly respected colleagues had concluded it was something else. Perhaps they were right and I needed to look at Phirun from a different vantage point. In one sense, I already had: I had told Phirun and his wife at the first visit that if this was a new condition, it would likely be the autoimmune disorder polymyalgia rheumatica (PMR).

My other concern was the craniopharyngioma. Was the remnant of that cyst somehow in play? His thyroid function was about 50 percent of normal, and his cortisol level was also suppressed. But the radiologist I consulted to review the brain MRI concluded that the remaining portion of the cyst was unlikely to be the cause of Phirun's problems. To discuss the case further, we assembled an ad hoc think tank — the chief resident Dr. Lee Fidler and two fourth-year residents, Dr. Sean Leung and Dr. Patrick Darragh — and decided to treat with prednisone for an assumed case of PMR.

The response was almost instantaneous. Phirun could walk normally and his grip strength measurement went from 30 to

100. Phirun speaks no English, but when I saw him for the first time after this dramatic turnaround, he smiled broadly and flashed me a two thumbs-up signal.

I cite this difficult case to illustrate a potent symbiosis, the combination of high-tech in the form of sophisticated modern machines, and low-tech, the very human art of medicine. Both are often needed to reach the correct diagnosis.

IF WE DO IT RIGHT, the advance of technical forms of medicine can only serve to improve patient care and outcomes. But as specialization and subspecialization continues apace, it is also clear to me that the role of the general internist — a specialist with broad, multi-disciplinary knowledge and skills — will gain in importance. There will be many challenges in the years ahead, but I remain optimistic. I hope that this modest volume can inspire doctors young and old, specialists and generalists, always to seek the good in others, to help those less fortunate, heal the sick and not let even insurmountable difficulties stand in the way of heroic deeds. There is no greater joy than being your brothers' and your sisters' keepers.

Herbert Ho Ping Kong
Toronto
February 2014